Traumatic Incident Reduction and Critical Incident Stress Management:

A Synergistic Approach

Edited by Victor R. Volkman

Foreword by John Durkin

Traumatic Incident Reduction and Critical Incident Stress Management: A Synergistic Approach

Book number one of the TIR Applications Series

Copyright © 2007 Victor R. Volkman

Library of Congress Cataloging-in-Publication Data

Traumatic incident reduction and critical incident stress management : a synergistic approach / edited by Victor R. Volkman ; foreword by John Durkin.
    p. cm. -- (TIR applications series ; no. 1)
    Includes bibliographical references and index.
    ISBN-13: 978-1-932690-29-3 (trade paper : alk. paper)
    ISBN-10: 1-932690-29-8 (trade paper : alk. paper)
    1. Post-traumatic stress disorder. 2. Stress management. 3. Crisis intervention (Mental health services)   I. Volkman, Victor R. II. Series.
    [DNLM: 1. Stress Disorders, Traumatic--therapy. 2. Crisis Intervention--methods. 3. Stress Disorders, Post-Traumatic--prevention & control.   WM 172 T7776 2007]
    RC552.P67T7555 2007
    616.85'21--dc22
                                        2006029820

TIR Applications Series

- Traumatic Incident Reduction and Critical Incident Stress Management: A Synergistic Approach

- Children and Traumatic Incident Reduction: Creative and Cognitive Approaches

- Addiction and Traumatic Incident Reduction: A Person-Centered Approach

This new series from Loving Healing Press brings you information and anecdotes about Traumatic Incident Reduction and related techniques. Practitioners around the world use these Applied Metapsychology techniques. It is our opinion that stories of real-world experience convey the opportunity for healing that TIR provides. Readers interested in the theories behind TIR and Applied Metapsychology (the subject from which TIR is derived) should also consider the *Explorations in Metapsychology* Series from Loving Healing Press.

About our Series Editor, Robert Rich, Ph.D.

Loving Healing Press is pleased to announce Robert Rich, Ph.D. as Series Editor for the *TIR Applications Series*. This exciting series demonstrates the impacts of TIR and Metapsychology in the real world.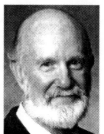

Robert Rich, M.Sc., Ph.D., M.A.P.S., A.A.S.H. is a highly experienced counseling psychologist. His web site www.anxietyanddepressionhelp.com is a storehouse of helpful information for people suffering from anxiety and depression.

Bob is also a multiple award-winning writer of both fiction and non-fiction, and a professional editor. His writing is displayed at www.bobswriting.com. You are advised not to visit him there unless you have the time to get lost for a while.

Three of his books are tools for psychological self-help: *Anger and Anxiety: Be in charge of your emotions and control phobias, Personally Speaking: Single session email therapy,* and *Cancer: A personal challenge.* However, his philosophy and psychological knowledge come through in all his writing, which is perhaps why three of his books have won international awards, and he has won many minor prizes. Dr. Rich currently resides at Wombat Hollow in Australia.

Table of Contents

Table of Figures

Acknowledgments

In order to successfully produce or even edit a book of this nature, the cooperation and contribution of many people is paramount. I would like to acknowledge (in alphabetical) order the following people who contributed articles to this book: Gerry Bock, Jill Boyd, Nancy Day, George Doherty, John Durkin, Frank A. Gerbode, MD, Robert Moore, PhD, Karen Trotter, and Carlos Velasquez-Garcia.

I would also like to thank the following people who contributed to the technical editing and proofing: John Durkin, Bob Rich, PhD, Ragnhild Malnati, and Marian Volkman.

Finally, I owe a debt of gratitude to the people who have made these techniques available to the world: George Everly, PhD and Jeffrey Mitchell, PhD, the International Critical Incident Stress Foundation (ICISF), the Rocky Mountain Region Disaster Mental Health Institute, Green Cross Projects, the Association of Traumatic Stress Specialists (ATSS), and the Editing Committee of the Applied Metapsychology International/Traumatic Incident Reduction Association.

This book is dedicated to all critical incident responders:
people who are prepared to put their lives on the line
every day to make a difference in the world.

About the Cover (clockwise from upper-left)

1. First Sergeant (1SG) Ray Gould, (left), USA, Military District of Washington (MDW) Engineer Company (Technical Rescue) and Airports Authority firefighter Liedke look over the damage on the inside of the Pentagons C ring. The hole before the men is where the airplane impacted. Camera Operator: SSG John Valceanu, USA Date Shot: 16 Sep 2001 (Released to Public)

2. Victims of the Southeast Asian Tsunami anxiously grab supplies delivered by a US Navy (USN) MH-60S Sea Hawk helicopter from Helicopter Combat Support Squadron 5 (HC-5), in support of Operation UNIFIED ASSISTANCE. DoD photo by: PH3 Rebecca J. Moart, USN Date Shot: 13 Jan 2005 (Released to Public)

3. U.S. Army Soldiers take cover behind vehicles and return fire on insurgents at a traffic control point on Alternate Supply Route Michigan in Tameem, Iraq, Aug. 16, 2006. The Soldiers are with Bravo Company, 2nd Battalion, 6th Infantry Regiment, 1st Armored Division, Baumholder, Germany. (U.S. Air Force photo by Tech. Sgt. Jeremy T. Lock) (Released to Public)

4. Rescue personnel from the Los Angeles Fire Department, the US Coast Guard (USCG) and the US Army (USA) search for survivors of Hurricane Katrina in a flooded New Orleans neighborhood. Rescue personnel mark a private residence, this ensures every house in the neighborhood is contacted. The Navy is contributing to the humanitarian assistance operations led by the Federal Emergency Management Agency (FEMA) in conjunction with the Department of Defense (DoD). (Released to Public)

Foreword

by John Durkin

It is an honor to be invited to write the foreword to a publication that addresses the two stress-interventions that have enhanced my personal and professional life immeasurably. Critical Incident Stress Management (CISM) and Traumatic Incident Reduction (TIR) have each led me to expect, rather than hope for, success in preventing and overcoming the debilitating psychological aftermath of traumatic experience. Each stands on its own as a practical and effective alternative to the isolation, avoidance and rumination of being left alone or being pushed to admit our reactions to a mental-health professional who may judge, label and medicate us.

This publication offers an extensive theoretical account of TIR, with consideration of why (or not) certain therapeutic approaches may be successful, courtesy of Dr. Moore's chapter. Nancy Day takes her experience of TIR into the world of crisis-response and identifies areas where those committed to crisis-intervention can benefit. Jill Boyd, a nurse who has been trained in both CISM and TIR, provides her unique view of how facilitation skills from TIR can improve CISM delivery. Karen Trotter shows how flexibly and confidently crisis-intervention can be applied in an extended and effective fashion through the Green Cross Projects, using examples from major disasters. These contributions explain how the approaches of CISM and TIR can complement and enhance each other.

Critical Incident Stress Management is a comprehensive system of crisis-intervention that employs peer-support for dealing with the aftermath of incidents that can have an overwhelming impact on those exposed to them. A short period of specialized training enables those with an interest in maintaining the mental-health of their colleagues to confront and address the emotional expression of their distress at the appropriate time. It is structured, phased and organized to facilitate recovery whenever an emotionally disturbing incident disrupts the ability to function. If you have not yet had formal reading or training on CISM, I would suggest starting with Appendix B, which reviews some fundamental aspects and definitions you'll need to successfully navigate this book. Similarly, if this is your first exposure to TIR you may want to start with Appendix A.

Traumatic Incident Reduction enables its practitioners, after a short period of specialized training, to resolve a range of distressing and disabling psychological symptoms. Following the Rules of Facilitation (see Appendix C) through an established protocol of repeated direction and enquiry, a rapid conclusion to even chronic symptoms can occur, often in a single session.

My discovery of CISM and TIR was the result of a search for practical and effective ways to deal with distress that came out of my own experience as a firefighter in England and as someone who was not helped by the clinical advice and treatment offered in the 1990s. I was retired from the fire service in England with Post-traumatic Stress Disorder (PTSD). I had been injured in a fall that saw me away from work for six months, during which time I became increasingly anxious about returning. Now, as a psychologist, I think I can see what would have helped me and why. I now train firefighters and paramedics in the crisis-intervention tactics of CISM and offer TIR training to the same people. Both groups of emergency workers are frequently and repeatedly exposed to incidents and scenes that can lead to PTSD and which puts them at high-risk for other trauma-related problems. I believe that CISM will soon be shown to be preventative for such problems and TIR reparative. While the academic and clinical communities argue about "effective treatments" and "evidence-based practice", I have witnessed nothing more impressive than watching anxious and fearful individuals piece together a new understanding of their experience to emerge, sometimes dramatically, with a renewed energy for their work and their loved ones. It seems to require no more than the safe-space that CISM and TIR can generate, motivation to stick at the task to completion and the discipline to follow the protocols.

The current advice of the National Health Service in the UK for people exposed to traumatic incidents is to allow a four-week "watchful-waiting" period, and to refer those showing symptoms of PTSD for cognitive-behavioral therapy (CBT), Eye-movement Desensitization and Reprocessing (EMDR) or drug therapies. The reliance on "experts" to deal with the effects of post-traumatic stress makes me uncomfortable. Reflecting on my own reluctance to approach or engage with a mental-health professional, I recall my belief that only a firefighter would understand what I was saying. Anyone who did not do the same job as me was unlikely to be able to acknowledge realistically what it could feel like. Additionally the outsider, no matter how expert they were in their field, was not an expert in mine. I even feared they might not believe me, or get upset or hurt by my vivid descriptions or judge me on dubious actions carried out when I felt I had no other choice. They might criticize, patronize or sympathize like non-fire service friends who wanted to know "what it was like" to attend certain incidents. Ironically, when I did seek professional help, I protected the therapist by pulling back from telling the whole story, only to realize that I was keeping them safe at the time I needed them to keep me safe.

If the most likely source of support in emergency work is a colleague, perhaps it is because they operate in the same space, share a culture and a language that is exclusive to the profession and tailored to the team; often they are referred to as "family". Not all families are healthy, but where justice, affection and equitable rules exist, there seems a good chance of a positive environment in which to operate. In a job (or a family) where safety is not assured, it takes the accumulated wisdom of history, insight and experience to survive and to function in a positive fashion. It is the wisdom, insight and experience of high-risk occupations that has informed CISM.

Critical Incident Stress Debriefing (CISD) was the forerunner to CISM and was first described by Jeff Mitchell in 1983. It was a formal procedure for emergency workers to meet under the guidance of a mental-health professional and a team of trained peers following a "critical-incident". Such an incident was one that might overwhelm an individual's normal coping ability such as the death of children, a colleague's suicide or a protracted, failed rescue. The emergence of additional interventions to add to the original CISD procedure (to become CISM) demanded a more flexible approach from its practitioners as crisis-intervention moved out of the meeting room to virtually anywhere a crisis-reaction might occur. Emotional reactions are not events that can be synchronized or predicted. Emergency responders sometimes recall significant parts of a critical-incident long after it has ended. Some will have aspects "stick" from the moment they are witnessed or felt and remain indefinitely in the form of unwelcome thoughts, images or sensations. An intervention should be available whenever an individual reacts and CISM is designed to do just that.

The limitations of the crisis-intervention tactics of CISM are acknowledged by being described as "emotional first-aid". The implications of the "first-aid" description are that crisis-intervention is likely to be brief, intended to prevent worsening and to promote recovery. Where significant improvement does not occur, referral to a higher level of care is demanded. With little more than a few days of training, it is assumed that crisis-intervention skills would not match those of mental-health professionals with years of academic education and clinical experience behind them. One crucial advantage of "peer-support" over referral to a mental-health professional, however, is access. Peers are not only familiar, they are available and likely to be familiar with the situations that have triggered difficult and painful reactions. Firefighters usually find something in the tragic that is positive, amusing or even hilarious and rarely, in my experience, do they ever seem worse for talking about it.

In her book *Trauma & Recovery*, Judith Herman identified three conditions that had to be satisfied before any progress toward resolution could be expected. She reported that *safety* was crucial, insisting that no recovery was likely without it. *Remembrance and mourning* could follow and then *reconnection* with people and what went before. This was the concluding stage and the best evidence of recovery. I have often compared that sequence to what I witnessed in colleagues in the midst of their crisis-reactions when no-one was available to provide the safety and therefore the opportunity to express what was remembered, what was lost and what it all meant. People in crisis are in fight/flight mode and cannot relax. They are therefore unlikely to find the time and space to piece together their experience, often fragmented, and arrive at an understanding of what actually happened and their part in it. No recall means no explanation and no explanation suggests that the job, the people or the world is not as predictable as previously assumed. When we sense a threat but cannot predict it, we seem to leave the radar on indefinitely. In CISM, a trained colleague is someone who is familiar with the landscape and can assist in realistically assessing the threat. Where this process is successful, the radar can be switched off and the energy directed toward more fulfilling goals than anticipating the next impact.

Crisis-intervention attempts to provide the safety necessary for the distressed individual to be able to remember and, if necessary, to mourn. If they assume it will be okay to say just what happened without hearing judgment, criticism or unfounded praise, they are more likely to express themselves fully than not. The crisis-communication techniques of CISM provide acknowledgement and encouragement as antidotes to the toxic effects of a crisis-reaction and seek to disrupt the development of a stress reaction in its early stages by handling whatever verbal or emotional expression is evoked.

TIR, with an emphasis on the skilled application of its Communication Exercises (see p. 139), offers safety in abundance. In my TIR work, I inform clients that "No matter what you have to tell me and however many times you have to say it, I shall still be here at the end." I trust that they believe it because I mean it, and it was what I needed to hear during the years I spent wondering where, and why, it all went wrong. The safety that TIR offers extends to the practitioner (facilitator) too. Facilitators in TIR are trained, drilled even, to put their attention on the individual facing them and to demonstrate their interest in them. With their focus on "the other", the facilitator does not attend to their own feelings on what is being said. To sense a visceral reaction to someone else's account is to become aware that attention is not any more on the client and to put it back where it needs to be, on the client. Many will recognize a transference process in that description and see the potential pathway to vicarious or secondary traumatic-stress for the listener. However, experienced TIR facilitators have questioned the existence of vicarious traumatization, which suggests that the transference pathway may be blocked or unavailable through TIR, and this protects a practitioner from such effects. Add to that the expectation of a positive, and often dramatic, outcome and there seems little for the TIR facilitator to be vicariously traumatized by.

The authors of the following chapters appear to have recognized the qualities of each approach and the "greater whole" that they create together. In his chapter, Carlos Velasquez uses CISD as an example of a crisis-intervention technique within CISM that matches the goal of TIR in verbalizing experience in order to generate meaning. He points out that the individual is at the heart of both processes with the procedure providing the structure and direction that enables those who may otherwise be reluctant to speak to do so.

Gerry Bock, with his experience in the mental-health field, shows how the principles of CISM can be applied flexibly enough to allow TIR techniques to be implemented, and to bring those techniques to finish whatever emotional work a CISM intervention starts. It is assumed in CISM that the problem of an unresolved crisis-reaction lies in the domain of psychotherapy and is beyond the scope of peer-support. I believe that TIR challenges that assumption, as Gerry Bock suggests, and can assist a rapid and lasting recovery, especially if the appropriate mental-health resources are impoverished or unavailable. Like CISM, TIR can be learned through a short specialized training program and improved with ongoing supervision.

While the crisis-intervention community considers whether TIR can meet the demands of the referral role that CISM rules demand, Carlos Velasquez and Nancy Day strike a similar philosophical note in identifying TIR as a person-centered model, rather than a medical model of intervention; a cursory examination of CISM will show it too is person-centered in its approach. Both point to the detailed and extensive communication work involved in TIR training. Each sees that the ability to employ its enhanced communication skills will equip those involved in CISM with greater sensitivity and enable them to work to greater effect. It may be that with TIR-trained peers in the CISM team, there is an answer to the perennial question,

"Who debriefs the debriefers?" The answer is: anyone trained in TIR.

TIR offers an opportunity for the members of a CISM team to deal with any accumulated emotional baggage that their involvement in crisis-intervention has created. Training in TIR adds another tool to the toolkit of crisis-intervention techniques and enables peer-support to address an extended range of crisis-reactions, even those that might justify a clinical diagnosis. If virtually all the emotional reactions of a colleague in crisis could be accommodated and addressed through CISM and TIR, then the difference to the individual, the CISM team and the community would be immense. I look forward to the day that what practitioners of CISM and TIR already know is recognized in order for these approaches to be embraced and enjoyed more widely. For those already trained in either CISM or TIR and do not yet know the other, I look forward to hearing how your practice is enhanced by learning from the other discipline. I expect the contribution of the authors of this publication will go a long way in assisting that to happen.

John Durkin.
August 11th, 2006

1

TIR As a Companion to Critical Incident Stress Management & Debriefing

By Nancy L. Day, CTS, CTM

[Ed. Note: this set of two papers was originally presented in the Proceedings of the Rocky Mountain Region Disaster Mental Health Institute's annual conference in 2005.]

Robert H. Moore, Ph.D. wrote *Traumatic Incident Reduction: Primary Resolution of the Post-Traumatic Stress Disorder*, the article which follows this introduction, in 1992. He has been a staunch supporter of Traumatic Incident Reduction (TIR) from its development in the mid-1980s, when he and TIR's developer, psychiatrist Frank A. Gerbode, M.D., introduced it to mental health professionals here in the US and abroad.

Even though there are trained TIR facilitators in Canada, Europe, South Africa, Israel and Australia, there are still too few, even here in the US, to meet the demand for skilled trauma rehabilitation services. It is my hope that Dr. Moore's article will inspire you to consider becoming trained as a TIR facilitator yourself. As a crisis responder, you doubtless will see many opportunities to use TIR's uniquely efficient and effective clinical protocol, not only to restore trauma victims to full functionality but to facilitate their subsequent personal growth.

What Dr. Moore does not mention specifically in his article is where TIR fits in with Critical Incident Stress Management and Debriefing; that is what I most want to address in this introduction.

Dr. Gerbode's purpose in developing TIR was to put into the hands of any caring and competent helper a structured technique for completely resolving PTSD, its sequelae and other trauma-related disorders. The technique had to be easy to teach, easy to learn, as well as highly effective in a short period of time. And he succeeded beyond all reasonable expectations. TIR's integrative and thoroughly client- or person-centered protocol fulfills the promise and is uniquely appropriate for use by lay practitioners as well as by mental health professionals. It is now the core procedure of "Applied Metapsychology."

Metapsychology facilitators neither interpret nor judge people's behavior and beliefs. Nor do they label them. They simply help people rid themselves of their personal anguish with a systematic approach to personal development that draws upon the common elements of human experience. They offer a practical, cross-culturally applicable program for self-improvement based on an understanding of the ways in which habits, reactions, attitudes and their associated mental "baggage" are acquired.

Whereas traditional psychology focuses mainly on reconstructing cognition, emotion and behavior, Metapsychology addresses internalized pain, confusion and thwarted intentions. The cumulative impact of life's mishaps, abuses, over-control, losses and deprivations is often expressed as negative personality and character traits. Applied Metapsychology identifies such mishaps and abuses, resolves them and revises the otherwise destructive pattern of failed coping and compensation that so often sabotages the best efforts of those who already have been injured or victimized. The result: a person who is truly and spontaneously happy and productive, a victim no more.

As you know, recovery is the longest phase in getting back to normal following a crisis... not only after area-wide events, like the recent tsunami or the hurricane that struck New Orleans, but when someone has endured a personal tragedy. CISM responders see it all. They do a tremendous job in supporting individuals during and immediately following both personal crises and large-scale disasters. But what happens to the victims in need of follow-up after the crisis has passed and the CISM teams leave? And how do CISM team members handle secondary trauma and support each other?

Crisis responders need to be able to recover quickly both to maintain a sense of normalcy in their lives and to be ready to respond to the next crisis. And they need to be able to return to their families confident that the people they have briefly helped will get whatever additional help and support they need to normalize or adapt. This is where TIR shines.

It would be ideal if every crisis responder could resolve his or her own past traumas before engaging in crisis work. More realistically, an effective crisis responder will have the ability to function proficiently even when he personally has experienced a negative reaction during deployment. The ability to remain "grounded" and functional in a crisis is strengthened by TIR training, as are communication skills. At no other time are the clarity and presence of mind typical of a trained TIR facilitator more vital than when a crisis has thrown others into disarray. As critical incident responders, we need to have our wits about us. TIR training gives us the opportunity.

Critical Incident Stress Management & Debriefing units that include well-trained TIR facilitators are better equipped to provide the kind of follow-up service that both victims and responders sometimes need after the crisis has passed. As a TIR facilitator, a CISM team member's effectiveness in relieving traumatic stress and resolving PTSD is greatly enhanced.

To find out when and where your nearest TIR professional skills workshop is being presented or to arrange for the TIR workshop to be presented at your facility, you are invited to visit www.TIRTraining.org.

TIR: Primary Resolution of the Post–Traumatic Stress Disorder

Robert H. Moore, Ph.D.

[Ed. Note: This is an adaptation of a book chapter introducing Traumatic Incident Reduction[1]. This chapter is not a guide to clinical application of the procedure nor is a training manual per se. Regardless of one's prior training and experience, we feel that successful clinical application of TIR requires a minimum of four days of training plus a brief supervised internship.]

Problem Profile

In recent years, significant media attention has been given to the Post-Traumatic Stress Disorders (PTSD) of Vietnam veterans, whose post-war "nervous" problems (i.e., sleep disturbances, hypervigilance, paranoia, panic attacks, explosive rages and intrusive thoughts) were known to veterans of earlier campaigns as "battle fatigue," "shell shock," and "war neurosis" (Kelly, 1985). As any number of mugging, rape, and accident victims have demonstrated, however, one need not have been a casualty of war to experience the problem (APA, 1987). PTSD appears in children as well as adults (Eth & Pynoos, 1985) and has been attributed to abuse, abortions, burns, broken bones, surgery, rape, overwhelming loss, animal attacks, drug overdoses, near-drownings, bullying, intimidation and similar traumata.

The PTSD reaction is most easily distinguished from emotional problems of other sorts by its signature flashback: the involuntary and often agonizing recall of a past traumatic incident. It can be triggered by an almost limitless variety of present cognitive and perceptual cues

(Kilpatrick, 1985; Foa, 1989). Lodged like a startle response beyond conscious control, the reaction frequently catapults its victims into a painful dramatization of an earlier trauma and routinely either distorts or eclipses their perception of present reality. Although we can't confirm that any of the countless animal species with which researchers have replicated Pavlov's (1927) conditioned response ever actually flashed back to their acquisition experiences, the mechanism of classical conditioning is apparent in every case of PTSD. As salivation is to Pavlov's dog, so PTSD is to its victims.

Like emotional problems of other sorts, however, PTSD is not accounted for solely in terms of antecedent trauma and classical conditioning. In order to provoke a significant stress reaction, as Ellis (1962) and others observe, an experience must ordinarily stimulate certain components of an individual's pre-existing belief system. Veronen and Kilpatrick (1983) confirm that the rule holds for trauma as well as for more routine experience. Errant beliefs—related to the tolerance of discomfort and distress; beliefs about performance, approval, and self-worth; and how others should behave—"may be activated by traumatic events and lead to greater likelihood of developing and maintaining PTSD symptomatology and other emotional reactions. Individuals who premorbidly hold such beliefs in a dogmatic and rigid fashion are at greater risk of developing PTSD and experiencing more difficulty coping with the resulting PTSD symptomatology" (Warren & Zgourides, 1991, p. 151). Also activated and often shattered by trauma are assumptions regarding personal invulnerability; a world that is meaningful, comprehensible, predictable and just; and the trustworthiness of others (Janoff-Bulman, 1985; Roth & Newman, 1991). Such pre-existing beliefs and assumptions, plus the various conclusions, decisions and attitudes specific to a particular traumatic incident (especially when held as imperatives) constitute the operant cognitive components of PTSD.

PTSD is as diverse in its symptomatic expression as in its experiential origin (see Table 1-1). It manifests as a wide range of anxieties, insecurities, phobias, panic disorders, anger and rage reactions, guilt complexes, mood and personality anomalies, depressive reactions, self-esteem problems, somatic complaints, and compulsions (Dansky et al, 1990). Because of the considerable breadth of its symptomatology, "PTSD" alone does not constitute a fully adequate diagnosis. The current PTSD-related diagnostic lexicon allows us to designate a case only as either chronic/delayed or acute (APA, 1987). It does not enable us to communicate either the specific features or the psychodynamics of a case. Assuming, for example, that a telltale flashback or some other clinical indicator properly identified them, each of the following case presentations could easily qualify as PTSD:

- The father who explodes in violent rages at his two year-old's spills and messes (combat veteran with delayed onset PTSD)

- The graduate student who gets so panicky at exams and interviews that he can barely function (severe childhood sports injury)

- The housewife who is bored to tears by her dull routine but can't get motivated to start a new activity (physically abused as a child)

- The college co-ed who desperately makes and breaks love relationships at the rate of three or four a semester (date-raped in her teens)

- The ten year old who gets nauseated and faint at the mere suggestion that he get into a car (parents killed in an auto accident)

**TABLE 1-1: Diagnostic criteria for
309.89 Post-Traumatic Stress Disorder**

A. The person has experienced an event that is outside the range of usual human experience and that would be markedly distressing to almost anyone, e.g., serious threat to one's life or physical integrity; serious threat or harm to one's children, spouse, or other close relatives and friends; sudden destruction of one's home or community; or seeing another person who has recently been, or is being, seriously injured or killed as the result of an accident or physical violence.

B. The traumatic event is persistently re-experienced in at least one of the following ways:

(1) recurrent and intrusive distressing recollections of the event (in young children, repetitive play in which themes or aspects of the trauma are expressed)

(2) recurrent distressing dreams of the event

(3) sudden acting or feeling as if the traumatic event were recurring (includes a sense of reliving the experience, illusions, hallucinations, and dissociative [flashback] episodes, even those that occur upon awakening or when intoxicated)

(4) intense psychological distress at exposure to events that symbolize or resemble an aspect of the traumatic event, including anniversaries of the trauma

C. Persistent avoidance of stimuli associated with the trauma or numbing of general responsiveness (not present before the trauma), as indicated by at least three of the following:

(1) efforts to avoid thoughts or feelings associated with the trauma

(2) efforts to avoid activities or situations that arouse recollections of the trauma

(3) inability to recall an important aspect of the trauma (psychogenic amnesia)

(4) markedly diminished interest in significant activities (in young children, loss of recently acquired developmental skills such as toilet training or language skills)

(5) feeling of detachment or estrangement from others

(6) restricted range of affect, e.g., unable to have loving feelings

(7) sense of a foreshortened future, e.g., does not expect to have a career, marriage, or children, or a long life

D. Persistent symptoms of increased arousal (not present before the trauma), as indicated by at least two of the following:

(1) difficulty falling or staying asleep

(2) irritability or outbursts of anger

(3) difficulty concentrating

(4) hypervigilance

(5) exaggerated startle response

(6) physiologic reactivity upon exposure to events that symbolize or resemble an aspect of the traumatic event (e.g., a woman who was raped in an elevator breaks out in a sweat when entering any elevator)

E. Duration of the disturbance (symptoms in B, C, and D) of at least one month.

Specify delayed onset if the onset of symptoms was at least six months after the trauma

Reprinted with permission from the *Diagnostic and Statistical Manual of Mental Disorders, 3rd Ed.,* Revised. Copyright 1987 American Psychiatric Association

The designation "PTSD," then, is not associated with any particular symptom, symptom cluster, or stressful current circumstance but denotes, instead, the historic mechanism by which any of a broad range of conditioned responses, along with their cognitive structures were incorporated into a client's repertoire.

Primary and Secondary Trauma

What makes PTSD a particularly persistent and pernicious variety of disturbance is the occurrence, at the time of its acquisition trauma, of significant physical and/or emotional pain. Such pain, in association with the other perceptual stimuli, thoughts, and feelings one experiences at the time, constitutes the "primary" traumatic incident. The composite memory of the primary incident, therefore, contains not only the dominant audio/visual impressions of that moment, but also one's mind-set (motives, purposes, intentions) and visceral (emotional and somatic) reactions. Thus, whenever one subsequently encounters a "restimulator" —any present-time sensory, perceptual, cognitive, or emotive stimulus similar to one of those contained in the memory of an earlier trauma—one is likely to be consciously or unconsciously "reminded" of and, therefore, to re-activate its associated pain or upset. It is this subsequent painful reminder, the involuntary "restimulation" of the primary trauma, that constitutes the painful secondary experience we recognize as PTSD (Foa, 1989).

In the Pavlovian model, the occurrence of the restimulator (triggering stimulus) equates to the ringing of the bell; the stress reaction itself equates to salivation. The mechanism is almost indefinitely extendible by association. Once the dog has been conditioned to salivate to the ringing of the bell, for example, the bell may be paired with a new perceptual stimulus—say, the flashing of a light—so that the dog will then salivate to the light as well as to the bell. If one next flashes the light and pulls the dog's tail, the dog will learn to salivate when his tail is pulled (Hilgard, 1962). By sequencing stimuli so as to create a "conditioned response chain" in this manner, we expand the domain of stimuli that will elicit the salivation response[2].

Since the laws that govern the construction of the conditioned response chain in the laboratory are exactly those that govern the development of the post-traumatic stress disorder in vivo, this simple mechanism—the expansion of the secondary restimulator domain by association—has very significant implications for clinical practice. It is responsible for the longevity of many PTSD cases, for the persistence of PTSD symptoms in the absence of flashbacks (Moore, 1990), for many apparent compulsions (Goodman and Maultsby, 1974), and for the fact that any secondary PTSD experience can itself be restimulated and thus function as a traumatic incident (Kilpatrick et al, 1985).

This process may be illustrated by the following common example: A veteran originally injured in an artillery attack (the primary trauma) will often tend to be restimulated, even years later, by such things as smoke and loud noises. So it's no surprise when he panics, post-war, in response to fireworks. However, should he happen to be triggered into a full-blown panic reaction by a fireworks display while eating fried chicken at a picnic in the park, he is likely thereafter, as strange as it seems, to get panicky around fried chicken (whether he flashes back to the park at the time or not). In such a circumstance, fried chicken gets added to the domain of toxic secondary restimulators of his war experience, and the "picnic in the park" incident acquires secondary trauma status and is itself subject to later restimulation. If, for instance, fried chicken subsequently gets (or previously had gotten) associated with his mother-in-law (who prepares it for his every visit), his contact with her also becomes subject to PTSD toxicity by association. The dynamic effect of such repeated reactions over a period of time is a gradual increase in the client's toxic secondary restimulator domain. This, in turn, produces a corresponding reduction of his day-to-day emotional stability and an inability both to comprehend and to break out of his increasingly volatile reactive pattern (see Hayman et al, 1987).

The more reactions one experiences, the more new toxic stimuli develop. The more new toxic stimuli there are, the more reactions one has, which suggests that those experiencing PTSD would eventually come to spend most of their time with their attention riveted painfully on past trauma. In point of fact, that does happen. The longer and more complex the chains or sequences of secondary incidents become over time, however, the less likely one is to flash all the way back to the primary trauma. This is why so many PTSD clients who appear to succeed in getting their attention off their primary traumata nevertheless withdraw from many of the life activities they previously enjoyed. Because they flash back to "the big one" a lot less, their PTSD cases are presumed to have abated. In reality, such clients are in worse shape overall because a lot of little things in their traumatic incident networks (all the secondary restimulators or "cues" they picked up in the years following their primary trau-

mata) bother them much more than they did in the past
(Gerbode, 1989).

As neatly applicable as it appears to be, the basic Pavlovian mechanism does not adequately display the
cognitive aspects of the human conditioning experience as
manifest in PTSD (Warren and Zgourides, 1991). In fact, it
is the cognitive-emotive content of a traumatic incident
that distinguishes PTSD in humans from the conditioned
responses of other species. Gerbode (1989) points out that
some of the key cognitions contained in the memory of
any traumatic incident that later cause trouble when they
are restimulated are those specific conclusions, decisions,
and intentions the individual generated during the incident itself in order to cope emotionally with the painful
urgency of the moment. In such a circumstance, not only
would certain pre-existing beliefs govern one's reaction to
a traumatic event but also the traumatic event itself
would give rise to the formulation of new, potentially errant cognitions. Viewed in this light, PTSD is very much a
cognitive-emotive disorder and not nearly so simply Pavlovian as it at first appears to be. Accordingly, an effective
cognitive-emotive approach is called for in its remediation,
one in which the errant cognitions generated under the
duress of the trauma are located and corrected.

PTSD and the Cognitive Therapies

Secondary Approaches

PTSD is one of the few terms in the diagnostic lexicon
that reliably suggests the etiology of the disturbance to
which it refers. In so doing, ironically, it focuses attention
on an area that many therapists, particularly those with a
cognitive orientation, have generally chosen to ignore. In
actual fact, cognitive therapy is not entirely oblivious to
the historic roots of emotional disturbance and generally
acknowledges that stress reactions get programmed in

somewhere along the way. Dryden and Ellis (1986) point out that some emotional disturbance is directly attributable to such background traumata as natural disasters and personal tragedies. But recognizing that the cognitive processes responsible for a client's current disturbance are frequently preconscious and therefore accessible in present time, most cognitive therapists have traditionally favored challenging a client's current disturbance-causing belief system over directly confronting the earlier experience(s) responsible for its acquisition (Ellis, 1962, 1989).

Which of us, for instance, wouldn't tend to address whatever present errant cognition we could find that would compel an otherwise competent and loving father to whip his two year old child viciously for spilling something, instead of probing such a client's own childhood abuse for the acquisition of his punitive mind-set? And who among us hasn't employed a "counter-conditioning" relaxation or quieting routine to desensitize a client to the specific current social situation in which he invariably chokes up and can't speak? In so doing, we manage to avoid having to address the POW experience he flashes back to whenever he chokes up. Such clinical procedures, after all, are basic to the cognitive-behavioral repertoire (see Saigh, 1991).

Anxiety management techniques, such as Beck's (1976) cognitive therapy, Meichenbaum's (1977) Stress-Inoculation Training (SIT) and Lazarus' (1976) multi-modal approach, are similar in this regard. They combine the monitoring/stopping of automatic thoughts and assumptions, cognitive restructuring, and guided self-dialog with such techniques as covert modeling, role playing, relaxation, breath control, and various desensitization procedures. But the overall focus is nevertheless almost exclusively on a client's current (secondary) experience, cognition, and symptomatology (Olasov and Foa, 1987). The following "coping self-statements" used in SIT to deal with an anger-provoking situation reveal the present, situational/symptomatic focus typical of the secondary, reaction-management approaches:

> This is going to upset me, but I know how to deal with it...Try not to take this too seriously...Time for a few deep breaths of relaxation... Remember to keep your sense of humor...Just roll with the punches; don't get bent out of shape...There is no point in getting mad...I'm not going to let him get to me...Look for the positives. Don't assume the worst or jump to conclusions...There is no need to doubt myself. What he says doesn't matter...I'll let him make a fool of himself...Let's take the issue point by point...My anger is a signal of what I need to do...Try to reason it out...I can't expect people to act the way I want them to...Try to shake it off. Don't let it interfere with your job...Don't take it personally (Meichenbaum, 1977, p. 166-167).

A therapist's decision to focus an intervention mainly on a client's responses to day-to-day stressors is most understandable when the client does not report flashing back at the time of the upsets. Most non-PTSD clients, after all, have no special awareness of their early acquisition experiences and, therefore, have little or nothing to say about them. Their attention is fixed on a steady stream of disturbance-provoking current events for which both we and they realize they do need improved coping skills.

In the clear-cut PTSD case in which flashback is evident, the client not only puts the acquisition experience (the primary trauma) in focus right at the start, but also often seems virtually obsessed by it. Flashback content, which is often concurrent with the client's upset over something in present time, is so painfully "charged" that he or she is either barely able to shift attention from it or else must regularly struggle to resist attending to it (Solomon, 1991). In such a circumstance, the therapist who focuses intervention exclusively on the client's dramatic over-reactions to current (secondary) events (on the restimulator, rather than on what is being restimulated) bypasses the opportunity to address directly and resolve the core of the client's PTSD case. Such attention mainly to the present-time "cueing effect", according to Goodman and Maultsby (1974, p. 62), "explains many failures or partial successes in psychotherapy, despite the best intentions of patient and therapist."

Given the extreme volatility of the memory of a trauma, though, it's really no wonder that many therapists and their PTSD clients (tacitly) agree not to confront such incidents head on. To understand why this is so often the case, consider the following:

- It is nearly impossible to get PTSD clients to perceive or appraise objectively a traumatic experience they are in the midst of dramatizing.

- It is usually difficult, even when they are not dramatizing, to sell PTSD clients on the idea of re-evaluating a traumatic event that has given them nightmares for the last fifteen or twenty years.

- Cognitive restructuring, thought stopping, and stimulus blunting techniques give PTSD clients little or no control over their tendency to flash back spontaneously and go into restimulation.

- Helping PTSD clients minimize the disruptive impact of their intrusive thoughts and teaching them not to down themselves over the persistence of their symptoms is better than nothing.

It becomes understandable, then, that many therapists choose to assist clients in their ongoing struggles to distance themselves from the memories of their traumata in an attempt simply to limit the frequency and intensity of their post-traumatic episodes.

Therapists may actually bring superb therapeutic skills to bear on clients' over-reactions to a variety of contemporary stimulus-events (e.g., rage over a spill, anxiety at a meeting), but unless they help PTSD clients to resolve the prior trauma (e.g., auto accident, childhood abuse, war experience) that actively supports their current disturbance and to revise the errant cognition associated with that primary experience, they have elected not to address the PTSD at all. The result of such a purely secondary intervention is that clients' unresolved primary traumas continue intermittently to intrude into consciousness, and clients are left to struggle alone to secure a sense of rationality against the influence of these traumas.

Warren and Zgourides (1991) report that a combination of Rational-Emotive Therapy (RET), relaxation training, imaginal exposure to the trauma, *in vivo* desensitization to toxic external stimuli, behavioral rehearsal, and role-playing helped a PTSD client ("Eva," a sixty year old woman traumatized when a truck crashed into her house). Their report includes the observation that toward the end of her therapy, "Eva and her husband decided to remodel parts of their house so that less time would need to be spent near the part of the house where the accident occurred. This appeared to increase Eva's sense of future safety" (p. 163).

Eva's need to escape a persistently restimulative environment indicates that her post-traumatic stress response was still quite active at the end of her therapy. The report ends with this observation:

> "Even more debilitative than the phobic reactions to truck stimuli was Eva's difficulty accepting herself as more emotional, less confident, and no longer the rock of the family. RET

was helpful with this secondary disturbance. At termination of therapy, however, this problem remained an ongoing challenge for Eva" (p. 163).

This unfortunate and all too familiar outcome of an intervention too heavily focused on secondary issues is made more poignant by the following considerations:

- The client, although in somewhat better control, was actually terminated with her PTSD case still active (suggesting the therapist didn't know what else to do for her) and with no mention of follow-up.

- The client was encouraged to continue working on "accepting herself as more emotional, less confident, and no longer the rock of the family" (suggesting that she should never again expect to be less emotional, more confident, and once again the rock of the family).

- The authors chose Eva's case as most illustrative of the application of RET and related cognitive therapies to PTSD!

The acceptance of such a dismal outcome for PTSD clients is not confined to the cognitive behavioral domain. A report by Scurfield et. al. (1990) reveals a similar outlook at the American Lake Veterans Administration Medical Center Post-Traumatic Stress Treatment Program (PTSTP). According to Scurfield et. al.:

> It appears that a number of traumatic memories will never be completely or even perhaps mostly forgotten; after all, a number of war-related experiences truly are unforgettable. If so, it becomes imperative, then, for the veteran in effect to develop a 'better attitude toward,' and less toxic reaction to, intrusive symptoms. The development of such an im-

proved 'coexistence' with still continuing intrusive symptomatology seems to be a very
important and relevant stress recovery phe-
nomenon (and one that we teach in the PTSTP)
(p.198).

The indication here is that if a traumatic experience is
truly unforgettable (which most of them are), it must also
be permanently and painfully intrusive. This simply is not
the case. A fully resolved traumatic experience is neither
completely nor mostly forgotten. It is, by definition, simply
benign and incapable of intrusive restimulation (Fairbank
& Nicholson, 1987). But the message from the VA to the
veteran with persistent flashbacks, "You're just going to
have to learn to live with them!" couldn't be clearer. It
sends an unmistakable signal that some of our otherwise
competent and caring colleagues have not yet begun to
employ the more robust cognitive-emotive techniques of
primary PTSD case resolution.

Primary Approaches

Because a traumatic incident is, by definition, exceed-
ingly unpleasant, there is an understandable tendency, at
the moment one is occurring, to resist and protest it as
best one can. It is at just such moments of extreme physical and/or emotional pain, according to Gerbode (1989),
that one's thinking (evaluative cognition) is least likely to
be well-reasoned and objective and most likely to be irrational and distorted. There is, moreover, a subsequent
tendency to suppress and/or repress the memory of such
an incident so as not to have to re-experience the painful
emotional "charge" of its restimulation. Unfortunately,
suppression/repression of the memory of a traumatic incident effectively locks its distorted ideation and painful
emotion away together in long-term storage, along with
the incident's sensory and perceptual data. Thus, the
stage for PTSD is set. Fortunately however, when accessed
with the specific cognitive imagery procedure described

later in this chapter, a primary traumatic incident can be stripped of its emotional charge, permitting its embedded cognitive components to be revealed and restructured. With its emotional impact depleted and its irrational ideation revised, the memory of a traumatic incident becomes innocuous and thereafter remains permanently incapable of restimulation and intrusion into present time (Gerbode 1989).

It may seem a bit unorthodox to some therapists to assign more clinical significance to the cognitive structure associated with events that traumatized clients in the past than to beliefs associated with present events. If only PTSD clients' present disturbances weren't so tightly tied to and governed by their past traumata, we could forego such apparent unorthodoxy. The connection is inescapable, however, and neither orthodox (present-focus) cognitive therapy nor any other theoretical framework presently provides as thoroughly workable an approach to PTSD as one that directly addresses both the cognitive and emotive components of a client's primary trauma. Beck's cognitive therapy has a similar theoretical base. He refers to 'core beliefs', which may or may not originate in trauma.

Support for the necessity of dealing directly with the primary trauma to resolve a PTSD case comes from many corners of the profession. In their review of theoretical and empirical issues in the treatment of PTSD, Fairbank and Nicholson (1987) conclude that, of all the approaches in use, only those involving some form of direct imaginal exposure to the trauma have been successful. Roth and Newman (1991) describe the ideal resolution process as one involving "a re-experiencing of the affect associated with the trauma in the context of painful memories" (p.281). Such a process, the authors point out, brings the individual "to both an emotional and cognitive understanding of the meaning of the trauma and the impact it has had...and would lead to a reduction in symptoms and to successful integration of the trauma experience" (p.281).

References to the use of "imaginal" procedures and to the "integration" or "assimilation" of past trauma may also seem unfamiliar to the PTSD therapist who has relied mainly on those secondary or symptomatic approaches previously mentioned. Of course, we are not confined to the use of such approaches. Neither are we limited to addressing only the most immediately obvious and easily accessible components of our clients' experience. The cognitive structures they most need to revise, after all, are those which actually underlie their disturbances, whether such structures happen to be immediately obvious and directly accessible or embedded in one or more painful past traumata accessible only with an imaginal procedure.

For PTSD clients, in other words, there is a literal and clinically significant, trauma-based answer to the usually rhetorical cognitive therapist's question, "Where is it written?" Many if not most of the beliefs and attitudes that support today's PTSD reactions were "written" into our PTSD clients' cognitive-ergo-emotive repertoires during various acutely painful past experiences. This is what makes PTSD-related ideation so difficult to access and reformulate by ordinary therapeutic means. It is encapsulated, so to speak, in an area of memory that erupts like Vesuvius the moment the therapist (or anyone else, for that matter) so much as brushes against it. Only the skillful use of a specific cognitive-imagery process, at this point, can access and revise it successfully.

Additional support for the efficacy of cognitive-emotive imagery procedures is found in Beck's (1970) observation that "When a patient has an unpleasant affect associated with a particular situation, the unpleasant affect may sometimes be eliminated or reduced with repeated imagining of the situation." Grossberg and Wilson (1968) and

Blundell and Cade (1980) independently confirm that re-peated visualization of an anxiety-provoking situation produces a significant reduction in the physiological (Gal-vanic Skin Response) reaction to the threatening image. MacHovec (1985) finds that hypnotic regression can help a client to recall and revivify the trauma, permitting a venting of emotions and reintegration of the experience. Frederick (1986) maintains that a frame-by-frame imagi-nal review of a traumatic experience is essential to the dissipation of its associated anxiety.

Speaking specifically to the use of cognitive-imagery procedures in the treatment of PTSD, Warren and Zgourides (1991) report that:

> In fact, exposure is most often effective in fa-cilitating the types of cognitive restructuring described earlier. Keane et al's (1989) implosive therapy, Horowitz's (1986) gradual dosing, and Foa and Olasov's (1987) prolonged imaginal ex-posure are methods that help clients work through their traumatic event, discover and re-vise meanings, and develop more adaptive responses to the traumatic event (p.161).

It is important to note, however, that cognitive imagery and visualization procedures, including "systematic de-sensitization" (Turner, 1979), "flooding" (Keane and Kaloupek, 1982), "implosion" (Lyons and Keane, 1989; Stampfl and Lewis, 1967), "repetitive review" (Raimy, 1975), and "direct therapeutic exposure" (Boudewyns, 1990), are neither all alike nor all equally effective. Boudewyns (1990), for instance, describes Direct Thera-peutic Exposure (DTE) as "encouraging the patient to experience repeated or extended exposure, either in reality or in fantasy, to objectively harmless, but feared stimuli for the purpose of reducing (extinguishing) negative affect" (p. 365). Reference to its focus on "objectively harmless" stimuli identifies DTE as a procedure used here to desensitize a client to secondary (present-time) trauma. No such procedure should be equated with one that directly addresses primary trauma. Neither can any procedure that is confined to the fifty minute hour (as was the case in the Boudewyns study) be considered flexible enough to handle the average primary traumatic incident.

The cognitive-emotive procedure best suited to the task of thorough PTSD resolution must also accommodate the predictable complexities and specific peculiarities of a given traumatic incident network. As Manton and Talbot (1990) observe, "traumatic events...can bring into consciousness unresolved [prior] situations (with similar themes) such as incest, child abuse, or the death of an important person in the victim's life" (p.508). When clients have more than one trauma in their history, the only completely effective procedure is one that traces each symptom of the composite post-traumatic reaction back through sequence(s) of related earlier incidents to each of the contributing primaries. Interestingly, a very similar observation was made by one of our earliest colleagues, (Freud, 1984) who wrote:

> What left the symptom behind was not always a single experience. On the contrary, the result was usually brought about by the convergence of several traumas, and often by the repetition of a great number of similar ones. Thus it was necessary to reproduce the whole chain of pathogenic memories in chronologic order, or rather in reversed order, the latest ones first and the earliest ones last (p. 37).

The fact is that 1) PTSD clients generally have to work through some intense emotional and/or physical pain simply in order to get in touch with the thought processes associated with their traumatic experiences, and 2) the thought processes associated with their traumatic experiences control their current PTSD response repertoires.

Although we must wind the clock back to give PTSD clients the opportunity to confront the pain associated with their prior traumas, we have not abandoned our interest in remediating the errant cognition that controls their current disturbances in favor of some quasi-analytic or purely cathartic approach. The fact is that 1) PTSD clients generally have to work through some intense emotional and/or physical pain simply in order to get in touch with the thought processes associated with their traumatic experiences, and 2) the thought processes associated with their traumatic experiences control their current PTSD response repertoires. For these reasons, we remain as interested in seeing clients identify and restructure the distortions in their thinking about past traumatic experience as we do about any of their day-to-day concerns. As Raimy (1975) puts it:

> Many current therapies attempt primarily to relieve the client or patient of his pent-up emotion, either in cathartic episodes or over longer periods of time in which emotional release takes place less dramatically. If we examine catharsis more closely, however, we can readily discover several cognitive events which have significant influence on the experience. If these cognitive events do not occur, no amount of "emotional expression" is likely to be helpful (p. 81).

The simple fact is that in order to deal effectively with past trauma, we must guide the client through to its resolution in imagery. The imagery process itself, however, is just the means by which we help PTSD clients get through their residual primary pain. It is by revising the errant cognition associated with that pain that they are freed from the grip of their PTSD.

Traumatic Incident Reduction

The most thorough and reliable approach to the resolution of both long-standing and recent disaster PTSD currently in use is Traumatic Incident Reduction (TIR), a guided cognitive imagery procedure[3] developed by Gerbode (1989). A high-precision refinement of earlier cognitive desensitization procedures, TIR effectively resolves the outstanding trauma of the majority of the PTSD clients with whom it is used when carried out according to its strict guidelines.

TIR appears to be more efficient and more effective than other cognitive-imagery or desensitization procedures, as such procedures frequently focus mainly (and most often incompletely) on secondary episodes. By tracing each traumatic reaction to its original or primary trauma(ta) and by taking each primary trauma to its full resolution or procedural "end point" at one sitting (a crucial requirement), the TIR process leaves clients observably relieved, often smiling, and no longer committed to their previously errant cognitions. At that point, the traumatic incidents, their associated irrational ideation, and consequent PTSD have been fully handled, and clients are able to re-engage life comfortably in ways they might not have been able to do since their original traumata.

Done one-on-one, the core TIR procedure may be completed in as little as twenty minutes or it may require two or three hours (average: 1.5 hrs) of "viewing" per incident[4]. The therapist needs to be willing to take the time necessary to guide the client back through the relevant trauma, carefully following TIR procedural guidelines, to permit the client to work through the painful memories of the experience in order to restructure its cognitive content as needed for full resolution.

Ideally, PTSD clients correctly identify their active primary incidents during intake. Clients who have regular flashbacks generally do this with ease. Such clients may be briefed on TIR the same day and, if not on drugs, scheduled for viewing the next day. Their PTSD problems can often be alleviated within the week. It is not unusual for a TIR narrative procedure to resolve an "unoccluded" (obvious) primary traumatic incident in as little as two or three hours. Case resolution then would depend mainly on how many primary and secondary traumata needed to be addressed to restore full functioning.

More commonly, however, PTSD clients do not correctly identify all their active primary incidents at intake. A war veteran, for instance, may at first report with conviction that it all dates back to Vietnam; he's only had the problem since then, and that is the content of his flashbacks. Once he gets into it, however, he is sometimes surprised to discover that his wartime experience was actually secondary to some previously occluded or less memorable earlier trauma[5].

In chronic cases, including some phobias and panic disorders in which flashbacks are absent, clients often have no clue at intake as to where or when their reaction patterns were actually acquired. Although technically not classified as PTSD, many such clients have had a significant number of stressful experiences over the years. Yet they cannot, at first, identify any one incident as having been much more significant than any other. They are often thoroughly frustrated and discouraged, as well as genuinely baffled, about the persistence of their symptoms. Those among them who lead otherwise comfortable lives and seem about as rationally, day-to-day, as the majority of the population, frequently come to the usually erroneous conclusion that their problems must be genetic in origin ("run in the family")[6]. (Needless to say, such cases are not resolved within the week.) They are not generally a problem for TIR, however, as they may be handled to resolution very adequately by the thematic approach, a variation of the narrative procedure. Thematic TIR does not require clients to be aware of or to identify correctly the relevant historic components of their cases right at the start of their intervention. Instead, the thematic procedure simply traces each manifest (present time) emotional and somatic symptom (theme) back through its chain(s) of secondary incidents, one at a time, until the originally oc-cluded primaries come into awareness and can be dealt with routinely.

Toward clients' understanding of the TIR routine, which assuredly will be new to them, it is often useful to draw upon the illustrative value of the Pavlovian example mentioned earlier and with which they may already be familiar. One may point out, in this connection, that when the dog's salivation response to the bell (primary stimulus) is extinguished, the light (secondary stimulus) loses its restimulative potential automatically (Hilgard, 1962). Likewise, once a primary incident is completely resolved, none of the stimuli that had later become associated with it as secondary restimulators is capable of triggering any further reaction (Gerbode, 1989). This means that when the veteran fully resolves his "artillery attack" (and any other related primary incidents), he will no longer be vul-nerable to restimulation triggered by the various secondarily toxic stimuli associated with that experience. At that point, fried chicken and mother-in-law are back to representing nothing more than fried chicken and mother-in-law.

This may seem like a rather classical Pavlovian expla-nation, but one of TIR's main concerns is the ultimate correction of the PTSD client's trauma-related thought processes. With a little psycho-education, clients realize that it was the cumulative effect of their traumatic inci-dent networks on their cognitive-emotive response sets over a period of time that is responsible for the persistence of their PTSD symptoms. Then, once they understand that there is a way to shut down the networks' active components permanently, they'll be happy to use the TIR approach, even if you've already accustomed them to another technique. Then, even thoroughly frustrated and discouraged chronic and absent-flashback PTSD clients will begin to feel hopeful.

The lexicon of TIR reflects its purpose and procedure. The client is called a "viewer" because his/her primary function is to confront past trauma via the viewing process. The person conducting the session is called a "facilitator" because his/her purpose is simply to facilitate the viewer's process of viewing (Gerbode, 1989). Just as "physician" and "patient" become "analyst" and "analysand" or "surgeon" and "organ donor," based on the requirements of their respective roles, the designations "facilitator" and "viewer" are reserved for those whose interaction is governed by the singular requirements of the TIR process.

TIR, like other cognitive-imagery processes, differs somewhat from most contemporary therapies. Although it holds errant cognition to be at the root of emotional disturbance, unlike the mainstream cognitive approaches, TIR carries the revision process back to the specific experience(s) that originally produced and enforced such cognition. In this regard, TIR is a bit more "personal" than most contemporary cognitive therapies. Instead of relying mainly upon the therapist's insight into or inferences about a client's probable belief structure, as is common for instance in RET, TIR guides clients in the discovery and revision of their own original disturbance-causing cognitions.

What makes such a procedure both necessary and possible is the fact that, in PTSD, the disturbance-causing cognitions (except for the pre-existing ones) were originally generated in response to, and in order to cope with, a traumatically painful and/or upsetting experience. Moreover, the offending cognitions are still being kept in force by the long-term residual impact of the incident. In other words, if it hadn't been for the specific circumstance of the trauma, as subjectively experienced by the client, e.g., "Oh my God, I've been shot! I'm gonna die!", the client wouldn't have formulated the response, e.g., "I should never let my guard down, even for a minute!" Moreover, if the incident hadn't been so emotionally and/or physically painful, making it extremely difficult for the client to confront, its attendant cognition would be a great deal more accessible to routine reappraisal and restructuring.

So, while it remains very useful to be able to infer with reasonable certainty that an anxious client is generally feeling threatened and ineffectual while an angry client would like to assert control over something (pardon the reductionism), these are just some of the more obvious "common denominator" dynamics associated with their respective current disturbances. What we cannot infer, but what TIR reveals to clients who have experienced trauma, is exactly what happened (at a subjective/cognitive-emotive level) that so overwhelmed them that they came away from their experience stuck in an involuntary, out-of-date, and irrational mind-set constructed, among other things, of numerous fairly obvious stress-producing mis-evaluations and distortions.

In a certain respect, TIR adds a new dimension to our understanding of the relationship between cognition and emotion. While theorists have long held that irrational and distorted thinking tends to promote upset feelings, TIR suggests that one's (traumatically) upset feelings also tend to promote irrational and distorted thinking. Dodging the "Which came first?" (chicken or egg) question, it is probably safe to say that, on the face of it, the causal equation appears to be reversible. That is, not only does cognition significantly influence emotion but emotion appears to significantly influence cognition.

Even more critically significant, at least in cases of PTSD, the remedial equation seems to be reversible as well. Whereas cognitive therapists observe that the restructuring of one's irrational and distorted thinking produces a corresponding reduction of emotional disturbance, TIR confirms Ellis's (1990) observation that a reduction of primary traumatic emotional disturbance produces a corresponding restructuring of one's irrational and distorted thinking. In short, the client whose trauma has been fully reduced and resolved and who has become able to talk (and think) freely and painlessly about it (a TIR goal) almost immediately and self-directedly begins to display a substantively rational (moderate, tolerant, objective) viewpoint regarding that previously painful experience. As always, the client who succeeds in embracing a more rational viewpoint about an experience, regardless of how unfortunate or traumatic that experience once seemed, is no longer disturbed over it or unwittingly under its control. As a consequence, secondary restimulation and flashbacks cease, life's energy and interest revive, and self-esteem rebounds[7].

What is particularly remarkable about the cognitive restructuring that takes place in TIR is that it takes place so obviously and spontaneously during the course of a given session. Equally remarkable is the fact that it takes place—and truly must take place— without didactic or corrective facilitator input. The facilitator's role in TIR is mainly to so conduct the session and guide the viewer in "repeated review" of the selected trauma (in strict accord with the established protocol) that the viewer will be able rationally to restructure his own "misconceptions" about it (Raimy, 1975). Bear in mind that at this level of intervention, the viewer is truly the only one who can decipher (by patient and careful re-examination of the cognitive im-

ages stored in memory) what actually happened or appeared to happen in the incident, what its significance
was, what he or she was thinking at the time, why it was
so extraordinarily painful, how he or she coped with that
pain, and what trauma-related conclusions and/or decisions were made at the time. So, as the viewer reviews
this highly sensitive and very painful material repeatedly
in imagery in order to discharge the emotional impact
holding the cognitive distortions in place, the facilitator
says not a word[8].

Although in TIR's handling of PTSD, the operant
trauma-related distortions virtually self-correct once the
inordinate emotional distress of the traumatic experience
is relieved, viewers frequently want to follow a completed
TIR session with some discussion or review of some of the
ways in which certain of their newly-surrendered trauma-
related beliefs and attitudes had affected them since the
occurrence of their original trauma. Most practitioners
find this discussion one of those truly rewarding moments
in clinical practice. It is not only confirmation of a successfully completed specific intervention. It is re-
confirmation of what contemporary theorists have as-
serted all along about the relationship between cognition
and emotion—with the additional suggestion that that relationship may be even more interesting than we had
originally supposed.

BIBLIOGRAPHY

American Psychiatric Association (1987). *Diagnostic and statistical manual of mental disorders* (3rd ed.), Revised, APA, Washington, D.C.

AMI/TIRA (2006). *Traumatic incident reduction workshop manual, 5th Ed.* Ann Arbor, MI: AMI Press.

Beck, A. T. (1970). Role of fantasies in psychotherapy and psychopathology. *The Journal of Nervous and Mental Disease,* 150, 3-17.

Beck, A. T. (1976). *Cognitive therapy and the emotional disorders.* New York: The New American Library, Inc.

Blundell, G. G., and Cade, C. M. (1980). *Self-awareness and E.S.R.* London: Audio Ltd.

Boudewyns, P. A., Hyer, L., Woods, M. G., Harrison, W. R., and McCranie, E. (1990). PTSD among Vietnam veterans: An early look at treatment outcome using direct therapeutic exposure. *Journal of Traumatic Stress,* 3, 359-368.

Dansky, B. S., Roth, S., and Kronenberger, W. G. (1990). The trauma constellation identification scale: A measure of the psychological impact of a stressful life event. *J. of Traumatic Stress,* 3, 557-572.

Dryden, W., and Ellis, A. (1986). Rational-emotive therapy (RET). In W. Dryden and W. Golden (Eds.), *Cognitive-behavioral approaches to psychotherapy.* London: Harper & Row.

Ellis, A. (1962). *Reason and emotion in psychotherapy.* New York: Lyle Stuart.

Ellis, A. (1973). *Humanistic psychotherapy: The rational-emotive approach.* New York: McGraw Hill.

Ellis, A. (1989). The history of cognition in
     psychotherapy. In A. Freeman, K. M. Simon, L. E.
     Beutler, and H. Arkowitz (Eds.), *Comprehensive
     handbook of cognitive therapy* (pp. 5-19). New
     York: Plenum Publishing.

Ellis, A. (1990). The revised ABC's of rational-emotive
     therapy (RET). Paper presented at The Evolution
     of Psychotherapy conference, Anaheim, CA.

Eth, S., and Pynoos, R. S. (Eds.). (1985). *Posttraumatic
     stress disorder in children.* Washington, D.C.:
     American Psychiatric Press.

Fairbank, J. A., and Nicholson, R. A. (1987). Theoretical
     and empirical issues in the treatment of post-
     traumatic stress disorder in Vietnam veterans.
     Journal of Clinical Psychology, 43, 44-55.

Foa, E. B., and Olasov, B. (1989). Treatment of post-
     traumatic stress disorder. Workshop conducted
     at Advances in Theory and Treatment of Anxiety
     Disorders, Philadelphia, PA.

Foa, E. B., Steketee, G., and Rothbaum, B. O. (1989).
     Behavioral-cognitive conceptualizations of post-
     traumatic stress disorder. *Behavior Therapy,* 20,
     155-176.

Frederick, C. J. (1986, August) Psychic trauma and
     terrorism. Paper presented at the annual meeting
     of the American Psychological Association,
     Washington, D.C.

Freud, S. (1984). Two short accounts of psychoanalysis.
     In J. Strachey (Tr.), *Five lectures on
     psychoanalysis* (p. 37). Singapore: Penguin
     Books.

Gerbode, F. A. (1986a). Assistance without evaluation.
     The Journal of Metapsychology, 1, 7-9.

Gerbode, F. A. (1986b). A safe space. *The J. of Metapsychology*, 1, 3-6.

Gerbode, F. A. (1995). *Beyond psychology: An introduction to metapsychology, 3rd* Ed.. Palo Alto, CA: IRM.

Goodman, D. S. and Maultsby, M. C. (1974). *Emotional well-being through rational behavior training.* Springfield, IL: Charles C. Thomas.

Grossberg, J. M., and Wilson, H. K. (1968). Physiological changes accompanying the visualization of fearful and neutral situations. *Journal of Personality and Social Psychology*, 10, 124-133.

Hayman, P. M., Sommers-Flanagan, R., and Parsons, J. P. (1987). Aftermath of violence: Posttraumatic stress disorder among Vietnam veterans. Journal of Counseling and Development, 65, 363-366.

Hilgard, E. R. (1962). *Introduction to psychology* (3rd Edition). New York: Harcourt, Brace & World, Inc.

Horowitz, M. (1986). *Stress Response Syndromes* (2nd ed.). Northvale, NJ: Jason Aronson.

Janoff-Bulman R. (1985). The aftermath of victimization: Rebuilding shattered assumptions. In C. R. Figley (Ed.), *Trauma and its wake*. New York: Brunner/Mazel.

Keane, T. M., and Kaloupek, D. G. (1982). Imaginal flooding in the treatment of a posttraumatic stress disorder. Journal of Consulting and Clinical Psychology, 50, 138-140.

Keane, T. M., Fairbank, J. A., Caddell, J. M., and Zimering, R. T. (1989). Implosive (flooding) therapy reduces symptoms of PTSD in Vietnam combat veterans. *Behavior Therapy*, 20, 245-260.

Kelly, W. E. (Ed.). (1985). *Post-traumatic stress disorder and the war veteran patient.* New York: Brunner/Mazel.

Kilpatrick, D. G., Veronen, L. J., and Best, C. L. (1985). Factors predicting psychological distress among rape victims. In C. R. Figley (Ed.), *Trauma and its wake.* New York: Brunner/Mazel.

Lazarus, A. (1976). *Multi-modal behavior therapy.* New York: Springer Publishing Co.

Lyons, J. A., and Keane, T. M. (1989). *Implosive therapy for the treatment of combat-related PTSD.* J. of Traumatic Stress, 2, 137-152.

MacHovec, F. J. (1985). Treatment variables and the use of hypnosis in the brief therapy of post-traumatic stress disorders. *International Journal of Clinical & Experimental Hypnosis*, 33, 6-14.

Manton, M., and Talbot, A. (1990). Crisis intervention after an armed hold-up: Guidelines for counsellors. *J. of Traumatic Stress*, 3, 507-22.

Meichenbaum, D. (1977). *Cognitive-behavior modification.* New York: Plenum Press.

Moore, R. H. (1990, October). Absent flashback/covert PTSD: a video case report. Paper presented at the annual meeting of the ISTSS, New Orleans, LA.

Olasov, B., and Foa, E. G. (1987). The treatment of post-traumatic stress disorder in sexual assault survivors using stress inoculation training SIT). Paper presented at the annual meeting of the AABT, Boston, MA.

Pavlov, I. P. (1927). *Conditioned reflexes.* New York: Oxford Univ. Press.

Raimy, V. (1975). *Misunderstandings of the self.* San Francisco: Jossey-Bass Publishers.

Roth, S., and Newman, E. (1991). The process of coping with sexual trauma. Journal of Traumatic Stress, 4, 279-297.

Saigh, P. A. (1991). *Posttraumatic stress disorder: A behavioral approach to assessment and treatment.* Elmsford, NY: Pergamon.

Scurfield, R. M., Kenderdine, S. K., and Pollard, R. J. (1990). Inpatient treatment for war-related post-traumatic stress disorder: Initial findings on a longer-term outcome study. Journal of Traumatic Stress, 3, 185-201.

Solomon, Z., Mikulincer, M., and Arad, R. (1991). Monitoring and blunting: Implications for combat-related post-traumatic stress disorder. Journal of Traumatic Stress, 4, 209-221.

Stampfl, T. G., and Lewis, D. J. (1967). Essentials of implosive therapy: A learning-theory-based psychodynamic behavioral therapy. *Journal of Abnormal Psychology, 72,* 496-503.

Turner, S. M. (1979). Systematic desensitization of fears and anxiety in rape victims. Paper presented at the annual meeting of the Association for the Advancement of Behavior Therapy, San Francisco, CA.

Veronen, L. J., and Kilpatrick, D. G. (1983). Stress management of rape victims. In D. Meichenbaum and M. E. Jaremko (Eds.), *Stress reduction and prevention.* New York: Plenum Publishing.

Warren, R., and Zgourides, G. D. (1991). *Anxiety disorders: A rational-emotive perspective.* Elmsford, NY: Pergamon.

About the Author

Robert H. Moore, Ph.D. (Clearwater, Florida) is an Associate Fellow/Training Supervisor for the Institute for Rational-Emotive Therapy (now Ellis Institute) and former Director of the Institute for Rational Living in Florida (1973-1990). He is Board certified/Diplomate in psychotraumatology (AAETS), a certified trauma specialist (ATSS), a Fellow/Diplomate of ABMP and IABMCP.

He has co-edited and/or contributed to six books by Albert Ellis and authored chapters on "Inference Chaining," "E-prime," and "Traumatic Incident Reduction" in books edited by Dryden, Wolfe, and Dryden & Hill respectively. His nationally syndicated radio and TV programs touched on various aspects of psychology for daily living. Now retired from his 30+ year clinical practice, he currently divides his time between corporate crisis management and clinical supervision.

End Notes

---

[1] Moore, R.H. (1993). Cognitive-Emotive Treatment of the Post-Traumatic Stress Disorder. In W. Dryden and L. Hill (Eds.) *Innovations in Rational-Emotive Therapy.* Newbury Park, CA: Sage Publications

[2] Since this classic example of the conditioned response is not of one energized by trauma, the magnitude and persistence of the salivation response will tend to diminish as the number of chain-linked secondary stimuli increases. The highly charged and painful PTSD response, on the other hand, demonstrates considerable strength and persistence through an almost indefinitely long chain of associated secondary stimuli.

[3] Emergency relief workers, paramedics, and trauma teams find TIR a highly effective procedure for use with survivors of natural disasters, violent crimes, and the like. It may be used as soon after the trauma as survivors are physically/medically able to receive it. It enables them to emerge from their ordeals without residual PTSD symptomatology.

[4] The actual length of a TIR session is dictated largely by the number and complexity of the incident(s) being viewed and by the ability of the viewer to confront them.

[5] Of course, some PTSD veterans are completely correct when they identify their wartime experiences as primary.

[6] Regarding the paradox of those who suffer emotionally yet seem to think just as rationally, day-to-day, as the majority of the population, and vice versa, Meichenbaum (1977) makes a provocative observation:

It may not be the incidence of irrational beliefs that is the distinguishing characteristic between normal and abnormal populations, (since) nonclinical populations may also hold many of the unreasonable premises that characterize clinical populations... The nonpatient may be more capable of "compartmentalizing" (upsetting) events and be more able to use coping techniques such as humor, rationality, or what I have come to call "creative" repression." (p. 190-191)

In this connection, it may very well be worth investigating the traumatic backgrounds of patient and nonpatient populations matched as to their incidence of irrational beliefs. Perhaps the unsuspected secondary impact of past trauma has something to do with the patient population's apparent inability to "creatively repress" the activation of their faulty thinking.

[7] "All theorists are faced with a dilemma in trying to explain how inappropriate affect can be severed from cognition. The same events can be interpreted as cognitive reorganization, as 'expression' of affect, or as extinction of a conditioned emotional response by nonreinforcement or counterconditioning. The cognitive explanation has a major advantage for psychotherapists in that its referents—the conceptions and misconceptions of the patient—are more accessible to direct observation (Raimy, 1975, p. 83).

[8] A complete outline of the TIR Viewing Procedure, basic and thematic TIR flow charts, the Rules of Facilitation, and a case illustration of thematic TIR in application are contained in Dryden and Hill's (Eds) 1992 book, *Innovations in Rational-Emotive Therapy*, published by Sage Publications, Inc., Newbury Park, California.

The book *Traumatic Incident Reduction* by French and Harris, contains a complete outline of the TIR Viewing Procedure. The first edition is out of print but a 2nd Ed. will be released in mid-2007.

Professional skills training in TIR is available in the U.S. and in other countries such as England, Italy, Canada, Australia and South Africa. The www.TIRtraining.org website is one place to find qualified trainers for TIR and workshops approved by Applied Metapsychology International, the certifying body for TIR facilitators and trainers.

(NOTE: The need for precision in application of TIR is such that a minimum of four days of prior clinical training in the procedure is strongly recommended. Said another way: we haven't yet seen anyone do the procedure successfully twice in a row who "learned it" from a book.)

2	# Critical Incident Stress Management and TIR
	by Nancy Day, CTS, CTM

[This whitepaper is based on Nancy Day's presentation given at the Northern California Regional TIR Conference on May 13th, 2006 – Ed. Note]

Jeffrey Mitchell and George Everly are the co-founders of the International Critical Incident Stress Foundation. They played a major role in developing a certain type of crisis response called Critical Incident Stress Management and Critical Incident Stress Debriefing. Their home base is in the Washington, DC area. They train people to do crisis response, and to teach others how to do crisis response the ICISF way. These are typically two-day workshops on peer counseling, group work, suicide issues, law enforcement issues and other focuses. Mitchell and Everly are the best known in the field for documenting techniques and developing courses for people who want to do crisis response work.

The main topic of my talk is where TIR fits in with crisis response. I do want to define what I mean when I talk about crisis[1]. Crisis is an acute response to an event wherein:

- Psychological homeostasis (balance) has been disrupted.

- One's usual coping mechanisms have failed.

- There are signs and/or symptoms of distress, dysfunction, or impairment.

---

[1] Caplan, G. (1961) *An Approach to Community Mental Health.* New York: Grine and Stratton;

Caplan, G. (1964) *Principles of Preventive Psychiatry.* New York: Basic Books.

One form of major crisis is a critical incident. This is any situation faced by survivors of an event, and by emergency responders who come to help, that causes them to experience unusually strong emotional reactions that have the potential to interfere with their ability to function, either on the scene or later.[2] Examples: a fire, violent crime, natural disaster, motor vehicle accident. Emergency responders include but are not limited to police, fire, ambulance, and evacuation workers.

Crisis responders and survivors both have varying levels of resilience. A lot depends on what our earlier experiences have been, and whether we have handled the emotional charge of the earlier experiences or not. Providing continuing education and training in crisis response and aftercare helps crisis responders to be more effective in helping people during and after the crisis, without becoming mentally impaired themselves. There is a large educational component to CISM, for people who are going to be doing crisis response as well as for potential victims. For example, some school systems prepare staff and students on how to handle a crisis situation. Even if a crisis never occurs in one's own school, being prepared is very helpful for warding off the symptoms of traumatic stress for staff and students who hear about incidents at other schools.

The definition of a traumatic incident, as Dr. Gerbode has said, is an incident that is partially or wholly repressed and that contains a greater or lesser degree of pain. Crisis is generally a trauma and a crisis is often very brief. It can be an incident that lasts just literally a few minutes or a person could be in a crisis for months, such as going through a divorce for example. TIR is a very efficient way of speeding up healing. People also seek this

---

[2] Doherty, George W. (2005) *Crisis Intervention Training for Disaster Workers Workshop.*

type of help when they tire of the pain from past incidents, or are actively avoiding stimuli or modifying their behavior.

Common Approaches to PTSD

- Coping Techniques
  - o Avoid situations that trigger past traumas
  - o Distract oneself when triggered
- Cathartic Techniques
  - o Release the emotional charge generated by past traumas, using methods such as psychodrama, implosion therapy, or focus groups
- Direct Exposure
  - o Controlled review of the traumatic experience in one-on-one session (TIR is in this category.)

TIR is similar in some ways to other direct exposure techniques. "Flooding" for instance is a controlled reliving of the traumatic experience. In Flooding, a "script" is composed by the client and the therapist and then narrated by the client in present time. "Flooding" is also applied to *in vivo* extended exposure, e.g. staying in a high place, looking down, until the fear eases.

As Dr. Gerbode says, "Trauma is pure receptive learning." The person receives data but because of pain, unconsciousness, or insufficient time, s/he is unable to integrate it, and the data becomes encapsulated as a trauma. TIR is an integrated learning technique. The purpose of viewing (what a client does in a TIR session, hence why he is called a viewer) is largely to integrate data s/he already has. The Rules of Facilitation and Communication Skills (see Appendix C), which a practitioner learns in the first level TIR Workshop, not only create a safe space and time for the client but also an environment in which integration can take place.[3]

Medical Model & TIR/Metapsychology

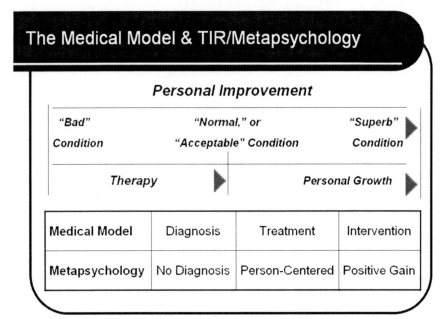

Fig. 2-1: The Medical Model & TIR/Metapsychology

I just want to mention briefly the differences between the medical model and TIR, which is a technique of Metapsychology.

Medical Model

- In the medical model, we have the "patient". There is a certain range of thought, behavior and emotion that is considered "normal" and "healthy". This can apply to both physical disturbances as well as mental and emotional disturbances. The therapist makes a diagnosis to indicate how the patient has

---

[3] *Traumatic Incident Reduction Workshop, 5th Ed.* (2006) AMI Press: Ann Arbor, MI.

departed from normal functioning. The DSM-IV very specifically documents what the medical profession considers not-normal or acceptable.

- The doctor or therapist then selects the treatment most likely to return the patient to normal or acceptable functioning. This is based on one of the neurological, behavioral, or psychological models of mental illness and its causes.

- The doctor/therapist then "intervenes" to treat the patient, thereby returning the person to normal functioning. Treatment may include drugs as well as therapy. When the patient's behavior, thought and emotion lie within the range thought of as healthy, the treatment is judged to have been a success.

- The treatment may create dependency on the therapist (for medication, client progress evaluation, emotional support, etc.).

Metapsychology (Traumatic Incident Reduction and TIR-related techniques and session protocol)

- In this model, we don't diagnose: the client decides which behaviors, emotions and thoughts s/he wants to change, and it is the facilitator's job to help the client change them. We're helping the client identify the current situation and ideal situation. Then it's our job as facilitator to move him/her closer to the desired situation.

- The facilitator does not diagnose from the outside, based on observation of the client, and there is no predetermined state of "normalcy" to achieve.

- As client, you are considered the authority on his/her mental environment. In viewing, the facilitator provides structure, and the viewer's mental and physical environment provide the context for the viewer to work. The whole ideology of viewing is structured to empower the client (viewer).

- What we are trying to do, as facilitators, is not to shift the client into any particular state of being or frame of mind, but simply to produce a change for the better, "better" being defined by the client.

- The techniques and session protocol empower the client and do not create dependency on the therapist or on viewing

- The techniques of Applied Metapsychology, including TIR, can be used to assist you to return to your normal state of functioning after something has happened to reduce the ability to function normally, and also to go past the person's old state of normal into an improved state. This work is in the realm of personal growth and development.

Timing for Crisis Response

Crisis response is done during the crisis or immediately following the crisis. For example, after the Tsunami, people didn't have any place to live; they were still looking for their loved ones, and assessing their own emotional status. Crisis responders can come in and start doing a series of briefings and debriefings to help people get grounded, so they can take care of the physical problems that they may be experiencing themselves, or sort out what they need to do to reclaim their property and so on.

Critical Incident Stress Management

CISM, according to the Mitchell and Everly Model, is structured into several interventions, which happen on a specific timeline and in this order:[4]

- Pre-incident Preparation
- Crisis Management Briefings
- Defusing
- Critical Incident Stress Debriefing (CISD)
- Additional Interventions for Individuals & Families

Pre-incident preparation is primarily education to enhance psychological resiliency in individuals who may be at risk of psychological crisis and/or psychological traumatization, by providing information and setting realistic expectations. This stage also includes specialized training for crisis response teams.

Crisis Management Briefings are a 4-step crisis intervention for large groups of individuals (up to 300 at one time) and is used in response to acts of terrorism, school crisis events, business and industrial crisis events, community violence, and mass disasters. The purpose of this briefing, which happens very early on, is mainly to answer questions. They give people as many facts as are currently known as to what took place and what the situation is now. For example, in industrial accidents or in schools after an act of terrorism, there are often large groups of people milling about or gathering in different places and they are in various stages of reaction. You can get those people together and just answer questions, to help them get more focused.

Defusing: A 3-phase, 45 minute, structured small group discussion provided within hours of a crisis for

---

[4] Mitchell, Jeffrey T. & Everly, Jr., George S. (2001) *Critical Incident Stress Debriefing*, 3rd Ed. Chevron Pub: Ellicot, MD.

purposes of assessment, triaging, and acute symptom mitigation (lessening). Triage is the prioritization of patients for medical treatment according to the seriousness of their condition or injury.

Oftentimes, when you hear of crisis response, you just hear the word "debriefing". The prior stages mentioned earlier (pre-incident through defusing), according to Mitchell and Everly, should not be called debriefing.

Critical Incident Stress Debriefing: A specific model of psychological debriefing. The CISD is a 7-phase, structured group discussion, usually provided 1 to 14 days post-crisis (in mass disasters, it may be used 3 weeks or more post incident). CISD is designed to achieve the goal of psychological closure and as a forum for psychological triaging so as to facilitate access to a higher level of psychological support. It takes small groups through different stages so they can express all the emotions and pain they feel. At the end of the 7-phase steps, the group is taken to closure or to a point of determining who needs more follow-up work. You can direct them to people like TIR facilitators who can help them after the crisis response people have gone home. Used for small groups of 4 to 25 participants, it is facilitated by the members of a CISD team, usually consisting of 2 to 4 specially trained crisis interventionists.

Additional interventions consist of one-on-one contact with individuals; pastoral crisis intervention; family crisis intervention; follow-up and referral mechanisms for assessment and treatment. Groups of people who are of the same religion or family can often be assisted simultaneously.

Naturally, with critical incidents and crisis, people are going to experience grief. Even if they don't lose a loved one, they might be losing property. Grief is just a process of working through memories and emotions associated with the loss of persons or property until an acceptance is reached that allows the person to place the event in the proper perspective. Some researchers object to the Kubler-Ross[5] codification of the stages of grief. I've seen the stages of denial, anger, bargaining, depression, and acceptance enough times to think that a lot of people do experience these stages similarly.

I am on a crisis response team in Kansas City and went with a chaplain to meet with a young wife and mother whose husband had recently been killed in a tragic accident, to offer her support, and referrals if she needed that. She greeted us at the door with a big smile, as if we were there for afternoon tea. She was clearly in denial. A couple of months later, when I asked the chaplain who was continuing to follow up with the young woman, if she was still in denial. He said, "Oh no! She's angry now."

Sometimes the various phases of grief can last a long time, but it varies from person to person. In doing crisis response, you need to be aware that some people, even during the crisis, may be walking around in a daze while others are racing around in a panic and others are being very heroic. You may see all the different phases right there on the crisis scene. The great thing about operating in a person-centered way is that we don't have to evaluate the condition of the person. We're not on a mission to "break" their "denial." We do need to be aware and to respond appropriately, and practitioners enhance those skills in basic TIR training.

---

[5] Kubler-Ross, M.D. Elizabeth (1969) *On Death and Dying.* Scribner: New York, NY.

TIR for Crisis Responders

CISM Steps	Does TIR Fit?
Pre-incident preparation	YES
Crisis Management Briefings	NO
Defusing	NO
Critical Incident Stress Debriefing	YES*

Table 2-1: CISM Steps and TIR Fit

*YES in the individual intervention stage in some cases and definitely in post-crisis follow-up and referral stage.

TIR is appropriate for pre-incident preparation. CISM provides education. TIR provides an opportunity for relevant personnel to handle their own mental baggage ahead of time so they can be more effective in helping others in crisis. People who may benefit include crisis responders, clergy, emergency medical technicians, firefighters, police officers and others who are called into action when a crisis occurs.'] Handling past traumas lessens the impact of the current crisis and thus speeds recovery. In summary, TIR for pre-incident preparation (for both crisis responders and potential victims):

- Eliminates mental baggage so that the negative energy and force of past traumatic experiences does not get triggered in life or in a crisis situation.
- Elevates communication and listening skills (through exercises in the TIR Workshop (TIRW).
- Enhances the ability to be fully present and to confront difficult situations with less chance of experiencing secondary traumatization.

For the crisis responder, as well as for *anyone* who is in a position where people are going to look to you for help, eliminating mental baggage and being TIR-trained is very beneficial and very appropriate.

For example, take the concept of triggering. Understanding how triggering happens is valuable data in itself for a person. Then he can say, "Oh, I'm getting triggered here," instead of just being overwhelmed by the experience and not being able to distinguish what's going on. You still may or may not know what is being triggered, but at least you can identify that triggering is occurring. It makes a person feel less crazy when reacting automatically, and more resilient when something happens.

Crisis Management Briefings, which go on while the crisis is taking place or during the immediate aftermath, are not a place for TIR. Defusing, which I talked about earlier, is not a place for TIR. As long as the person is still processing the trauma and still in the crisis, TIR is not really appropriate. But in Critical Incident Stress Debriefing, which I mentioned has 7 stages, the last of which is *referral*, TIR is appropriate and it is also a powerful tool for post-crisis follow-up.

TIR can handle the crisis responder's reactions, reduce secondary traumatization, and help the person to be ready to respond to the next crisis in a short amount of time.

For the individual who experiences a crisis and who doesn't get back to normal as quickly or easily as expected (or at all), TIR is a good technique for resolving the lingering negative aspects of trauma. To summarize, after the crisis has passed, TIR:

- Handles the responder's reactions to the trauma in a timely manner, before the next crisis response, thus preventing PTSD and compassion fatigue

- Provides an effective tool for following-up for trauma resolution (for crisis responders and for victims).

In a nutshell, TIR fits in pre-crisis and post-crisis but not during the crisis. It doesn't fit into crisis management briefings because that is done in groups. In a group, everyone would be reaching end points at different times and it wouldn't be manageable.

Recovery is the Longest Phase

After the crisis has passed, individuals may struggle in getting back to normal or a "new normal." TIR is an effective tool to help people with that phase, following a personal crisis or a community disaster.

As physical first aid is to surgery, crisis intervention is to psychotherapy.[6] Sometimes there just aren't enough mental health personnel around who are trained in trauma-resolution techniques. Sometimes people are reluctant to go to a mental health professional because of the stigma attached to being labeled with a mental illness diagnosis such as PTSD. This is particularly prevalent around firefighters, police, veterans, and people in the military. A mental illness diagnosis can affect a soldier's promotion and, for anyone, it may limit one's career options. Knowing this, people who really need help often don't ask for it.

Since CPR (Cardiopulmonary resuscitation) was first taught to lay persons in 1967, hundreds of thousands of lives have been saved by the techniques applied by them. Lay persons can also learn how to help their peers following a crisis or community disaster, using TIR and related techniques. TIR training is open to everyone who has a reasonable degree of intelligence and an honest and willing interest in helping people. Although I have a high percentage of mental health professionals in my TIR work-

---

[6] Everly, Jr., George S. *Assisting Individuals in Crisis: A Workbook, 3rd Ed.*

shops, I find that the workshop is really lively when there is a mix of both mental health professionals and lay practitioners; and people learn things they would have never had an opportunity to learn in a training environment of their peers only.

Children and Crisis

Children's perceptions of disaster or a crisis are largely determined by their parents' reactions or the reactions of other people they look up to. Research and literature suggests that children are generally more resilient and recover more quickly. However, they are still at risk for PTSD, depression, anxiety disorders and developmental delays. Parents who *respond* rather than *react*, in crisis and in day to day living, are less likely to create unnecessary trauma for their children. Improving one's mental environment where one can respond appropriately in any situation may be accomplished with TIR.

How Long Before Using TIR?

I know I've been talking about using TIR after the crisis has passed, but *after* the crisis has passed may just be a few days. It may not necessarily require waiting months. I'll give you a personal example of this. When my dad died, my mom was in the hospital with him and we didn't know that his condition was that serious. Mom helped Dad with shaving in the morning; he was on oxygen for respiratory problems. In the afternoon, she was just sitting there in the room alone with him and he was lying back resting. He rose up and grabbed his stomach, hollered, lay back down, rose up again, lay back down, his eyes rolled back in his head, and he was gone. I flew to Illinois that night and Mom and I were up all night. I was crying and she was recounting the traumatic event.

The thing that was most troublesome to her was that she couldn't remember if Dad rose up once or twice. She had repressed that part of the incident. That part she just kept going over... "I can't remember... Why can't I remember it? Why can't I remember it? So we got through the funeral and visitation afterward. A week later, I was helping Mom write out thank-you cards and she was still in the trauma saying, "I can't get this out of my head." So I said, "Mom, you know what I do. Would you like to go into session and address this?" We went into session for about 45 minutes and she recovered that missing part of the memory. Her awareness came up through the process of repetition. We came to a good end point with the TIR session and that put the incident in the past. I'm not saying that the grieving process was over, but Mom was no longer troubled by the incomplete picture. She never mentioned it again.

She was now ready to handle all the other changes she would have to make with my Dad gone. Even though my dad's clothes were still hanging in the closet and Mom had a lot of adjustments to make, that trauma was out of the way. This really greatly speeded up her recovery from the trauma I'm sure. Basically, if a person appears to be ready and is asking for help, I go forward.

Involuntary Reactions of PTSD

- Recurrent & intrusive memories
- Acting or feeling as if the trauma were recurring (flashbacks, etc.)
- Psychological distress and physiological reactivity on exposure to cues that symbolize or resemble an aspect of the traumatic event
- Outbursts of anger; exaggerated startle response; hypervigilance[7]

---

[7] *Diagnostic and Statistical Manual of Mental Disorders (DSM-IV-TR) Fourth Edition* (2000) by American Psychiatric Association.

Roughly 1 in 6 returning Iraq veterans suffer from PTSD, anxiety, or depression, according to a study by the Army that was published in the New England Journal of Medicine in July 2004. I'm told now that that number is much higher. Statistics consistently show that the best efforts of the military, VA, and other providers are not enough (by themselves) to prevent thousands of veterans and their families from suffering with homelessness, substance abuse, suicide and other psychological problems, incarceration, domestic violence, and parenting and employment problems, after leaving the military.[8]

A total of 53 suicides were reported among service members fighting in Iraq, and 9 among those fighting in Afghanistan, according to a review of suicide data[9] from 2003 to July 19, 2005. Most suicides, according to veteran groups and media accounts, occur after troops return home. For example, Marine reservist Jeffrey Lucey spent 5 months in Iraq, came home, was diagnosed with PTSD, and hung himself. On his bed his father found dog tags of two unarmed Iraqi prisoners his son said he had been forced to shoot[10]. I'm hearing as well from people I know in the military, that along with domestic violence, some husbands are actually killing their wives in the struggle to get back to normal functioning and regaining "control". That's something you might not hear reported in the media, but in speaking with an Army counselor one gets a better idea of what's actually going on.

I'm hoping that we can do something about the stigma of mental illness and make it easier for people to ask for help. It's also a fact that people who are not accustomed

---

[8] *Fact sheet*, Veterans And Families, 657 Brickyard Drive, Sacramento CA 95831; 916-395-4054).

[9] Hidden Combat Wounds: Extensive, Deadly, Costly". *Psychiatric Times*, January 2006.

[10] "Iraq War Veteran's Suicide - He was Swallowed by Pain", Mehul Srivastava. *Dayton Daily Times*. Oct. 11, 2004.

to, or financially able to, use outside help before they have a crisis are also not going to be willing or able to do so after a crisis. Unless there is a way to make it more affordable such as the Veterans Administration (in the USA), it won't be accessible.

Is CISD Effective?

There was some bad research done that said that the outcome of CISD was either ineffective or harmful. John Durkin, now head of the TIRA Research and Studies Committee, gives a very good talk about all the holes in the research that reported unfavorable outcome.[11] Based on my own knowledge and training, I believe that CISD/CISM is an effective method for helping individuals who have experienced major crisis.

The involuntary reactions of civilians with unresolved traumas may be similar to those of combat veterans. There are many civilians who suffer with PTSD, anxiety and depression, brought about by "normal" life experiences such as accidents, operations, divorce, job loss, major illness, etc.

Goals and objectives of CISD are:

1) Lessen the impact of the critical incident on those who were victims—primarily victims directly traumatized by the event; secondary victims (emergency services personnel); tertiary victims (family, friends, and those to whom the traumatic event may be indirectly communicated).

2) The purpose is to accelerate normal recovery processes in normal people who are experiencing normal stress reactions to traumatic events.

---

[11] Presentation at AMI/TIRA Technical Symposium 2004 at Goodenough College, London.

3) Identify individuals within the group who might be in need of additional CISM services or a referral for one-on-one therapeutic help.

This is accomplished through education, emotional ventilation, reassurance that recovery is likely and that victims' reactions are not unique but are normal. This is accomplished by establishing a positive relationship with mental health professionals, through enhancement of group cohesiveness and cooperation, through prevention or mitigation of Post-Traumatic Stress and PTSD, and by screening people who need additional help after the crisis has passed.

Involuntary reactions resulting from unresolved trauma include outbursts of anger, exaggerated startle response and hypervigilance. This can make life miserable for an individual and family. A constant "reaction" to outside stimuli feels like loss of control. People react to each other's reactions with a snowball effect.

While medication can help individuals cope with unwanted symptoms resulting from past traumatic incidents, it alone will not take away involuntary trauma reactions common with traumatic stress and PTSD. Clients often report that medication, as well as alcohol, actually cause PTSD symptoms to become worse.

No one who responds to a mass casualty event is untouched by it. Profound sadness, grief and anger are normal reactions to an abnormal event. Wanting to remain on the scene until the work is finished is normal. It is wise for crisis responder teams to have a self-care plan in place, one that team members readily accept and use. Peer to peer use of TIR would be a great addition to whatever you already have.

TIR is a technique that complements the work of crisis responders. In summary, here's how TIR fits in with the Critical Incident Stress Management model:

A) PREPAREDNESS: Critical Incident Stress Management (CISM) provides training to prepare people for crisis and for natural and man-made disasters. Responding appropriately in a crisis and adequate follow-up can prevent Post-Traumatic Stress Disorder from developing in individuals. Crisis responders who are not burdened with their own mental baggage will be better equipped to help others deal with traumatic stress. TIR is one approach to maintain balance in high stress jobs.

B) DURING THE CRISIS: TIR training heightens a practitioner's awareness of his own reactions and strengthens his ability to respond appropriately rather than to react.

C) POST-TRAUMA: After the crisis is over, and the CISM team has done crisis management briefings and debriefings, both crisis responders and victims who continue to be negatively affected by the traumatic incident will benefit greatly by using TIR to get back to normal as quickly as possible.

3

The Usefulness of TIR
in Training for CISM
By Jill Boyd, RN, MS

About the Author

Jill Boyd, RN, MS in Mental Health Counseling, works for the NYS Office of Alcoholism and Substance Abuse Services (OASAS). She is Director of the OASAS Crisis Response Team. She has taken (3) TIR workshops and numerous CISM courses.

Traumatic Incident Reduction

Once learned and integrated by a competent facilitator, Traumatic Incident Reduction (TIR) Rules of Facilitation and Communication Skills (see Appendix C) have many applications. One such application is applying them to Critical Incident Stress Management (CISM) tactics, namely, 1:1 crisis intervention; defusing; and debriefings known as Critical Incident Stress Debriefing (CISD).

To fully understand this application, it is essential to define the terminology. A TIR facilitator is a person who has learned how to enable clients to "view" the emotionally charged contents of their own minds. By doing so, viewers can get rid of the charge that has been making it impossible for them to control the unwanted and painful effects that the mind had had on them. (AMI/TIRA, 2006).

A facilitator follows a specific repetitive technique such as TIR or Unblocking[1] to achieve an end point of lessened charge on the part of the viewer. Although the steps are invariably the same, the content is person-centered in that the facilitator always follows the interest of the

---

[1] Unblocking is taught in the TIR Workshop. See also http://www.tir.org/metapsy/unblock.htm

viewer. Formally speaking, it is therapist-directed, person-centered, and non-hypnotic.

A viewer is anyone who, with the aid and direction of the facilitator, is systematically examining the contents of his own mind – his mental environment – in such a way as to gain insight and ability by undoing repression (AMI/TIRA, 2006).

Critical Incident Stress Management (CISM)

CISM is a comprehensive, integrated, multi-component crisis intervention system (Everly & Mitchell, 1999; Flannery, 1998). The core crisis intervention components of the CISM system are:

- **Pre-incident preparation:** this is a form of psychological "immunization" with the sharing of information that includes familiarization with common stressors, stress management education, stress resistance training, and crisis mitigation training.
- **Demobilization:** for a disaster or large scale crisis intervention which is a temporary psychological "decompression" immediately after exposure to a critical incident.
- **Crisis Management Briefing (CMB):** a 4-step crisis intervention for large groups of individuals (up to 300 at a time).
- **Defusing:** is a 3 phase, 45 minute structured small group discussion conducted within hours of a crisis for purposes of assessment, triaging, and acute symptom mitigation. Sometimes a defusing may foster psychological closure after a critical incident.
- **Critical Incident Stress Debriefing (CISD):** is a 7 phase, structured group discussion usually conducted 1 to 14 days post crisis. CISD is designed to provide psychological closure subsequent to a critical incident or traumatic event, or similarly serve as

a forum for psychological triaging so as to facilitate access to a higher level of psychological support.

CISD is designed to be used with small groups of 4 to 25 participants, although 8 to 10 is ideal. It is facilitated by members of the CISD team consisting of 2 to 4 trained crisis interventionists. Most teams utilize peers and have 1 or more mental health counselors present. Some teams have a chaplain present who is an active member of the team.

The CISD facilitator introduces the process in the *introductory remarks,* which is the first phase. This sets the tone, motivating participants to accept and cooperate with the format and establishes the rule for the discussion. The second phase of CISD is the *fact phase* in which participants describe what happened during the incident. The third phase is the *thought phase* in which the participants are asked about their first or most prominent thoughts at the time of the incident.

The fourth phase is the *reaction phase.* The participants are asked what part of the incident was the worst part for them. The fifth phase consists of inquiring what *symptoms* of distress which may be cognitive, physical, emotional, behavioral or spiritual were encountered either during or after the critical incident. The *teaching phase* is the sixth phase. At this time, team members provide information or suggestions on what can help to reduce the stress.

In the final phase, or *re-entry,* participants have an opportunity to bring up questions, concerns or other information. The facilitator *summarizes* the discussion in the seventh phase and closes the discussion. Team members are available for crisis interventions on an individual basis or to provide referrals for those participants who require further support.

- **1:1 Crisis Intervention** - is psychological support from 1 to 3 contacts with an individual in crisis.
- **Pastoral Crisis Intervention** – is the integration of traditional crisis intervention with pastoral-based support services.
- **Family Crisis Intervention as well as Organizational Consultation** – represents crisis intervention at the systems level.
- **Follow-up and Referral Mechanisms** - for assessment and treatment if necessary. (Mitchell & Everly, 2001).

Other terms defined by Mitchell and Everly in their *Critical Incident Stress Debriefing: An Operations Manual for CISD* (2001) are:

1. **Critical Incident:** a stressor or crisis event that appears to cause a crisis response which overwhelms a person's usual coping mechanisms. The most severe forms of critical incidents may be considered traumatic incidents.
2. **Critical Incident Stress:** a stress reaction a person or group has to a critical incident. Critical incident stress is characterized by a wide range of cognitive, physical, emotional and behavioral signs and symptoms. Most people recover from critical incident stress within a few weeks.
3. **Crisis:** is an acute response to an event wherein:
   - Psychological homeostasis (balance) has been disrupted
   - One's usual coping mechanisms have failed
   - There are signs and/or symptoms of distress, dysfunction, or impairment (Caplan, 1961, 1964).
4. **Trauma:** is an event outside the usual realm of human experience that is distressing to anyone experiencing it.

5. **Crisis Intervention:** is the urgent and acute psychological support known as "emotional first aid." The goals of crisis intervention are:
   - Acute Stabilization of symptoms and signs of distress and dysfunction and to keep things from getting worse.
   - Symptom reduction.
   - Restoration to independent functioning and successful reduction of impairment.
   - Access to a higher or more continuous level of care, if needed (Caplan, 1961, 1964; Everly & Mitchell, 1999).

According to Jeffrey Mitchell, who developed CISM along with George Everly, CISM is a "package of interventions, not an isolated tactic model applied outside the context of the overall strategy." (Mitchell, Everly, & Clark, 2006). In his article, "Characteristics of Successful Early Intervention Programs," Jeffrey Mitchell, states, "By no means is CISD the most frequently used intervention. In fact, it is more common for individual crisis intervention tactics to be used." (Mitchell & Everly, 2001).

Mitchell continues, "The primary function of a CISM program is to provide a range of crisis intervention support services to its target population. It is not a function of a CISM team to provide psychotherapy, medical treatment, legal advice, or 'cures' for any psychiatric condition."

The principal goals of a CISM team are:

- To reduce emotional tension.
- To facilitate normal recovery processes of normal people having normal, healthy reactions to abnormal events.
- To identify individuals who might need additional support or a referral to professionals for specific care. A CISM team provides "psychological first aid"

but it does not engage in long term psychotherapy. (Mitchell, 2004).

CISD and its parallel process, defusing, are group interactions initially developed by Jeffrey Mitchell for the prevention of post traumatic stress among high-risk occupational groups, specifically firefighting, law enforcement, emergency medicine, disaster response, emergency dispatch and public safety personnel. These processes have subsequently been adopted by the military, the clergy, the banking industry, airlines, and life guard services. The Employee Assistance Program (EAP) industry has begun to heavily utilize defusing and CISD as well as other processes. The earliest CISM teams were begun in fire and emergency medical services. (Mitchell & Everly, 2001).

Towards A Synergistic Approach

TIR Rules of Facilitation and Communication Skills (see Appendix C) can be successfully applied to many of the tactics of CISM, but mainly for individual or small group interactions. It is most helpful to think of the Rules of Facilitation and Communication Skills as a blanket of protection. Anyone who is experiencing critical incident or traumatic stress is in a vulnerable psychological state. Even though the mind protects itself by setting up defenses, once an individual is subjected to the material of the incident by viewing (or triggering), that state of vulnerability is reactivated. This may be become evident emotionally or behaviorally. TIR recognizes this state as one of carrying an emotional negative charge. Complicating the presence of increased vulnerability and negative charge are the inherent characteristics of the rescue worker, i.e. firefighter, Emergency Medical Service (EMS) responder, paramedic, etc. These individuals are highly dedicated to the task at hand. Their work gives meaning to their lives. It is a matter of identity with the self. Although the 7 phase CISD is not a critique and that is strongly emphasized in the introductions, rescue workers are their own worst critics. They blame themselves for any negative outcome as though it were a deficiency or poor judgment on their part. No matter how a CISD is conducted, facilitators will agree that most participants continue to hang on to self-recriminations.

Applying the Rules of Facilitation and Communication Skills are at the core of the person-centered approach originated by Carl Rogers, known as the Rogerian technique. All the Rules of Facilitation accept each individual without judgment and with an intention of helping. The art of the Communication Skills is readily discernible to the CISD participant. This is the difference between a seasoned CISD facilitator and novice. The experienced CISD facilitator is similar to the competent TIR facilitator. The individual has a "feel" for what is right and necessary for the group's healing to take place. However, the seasoned CISD facilitator has acquired those skills from many exposures to groups in distress. TIR facilitators, once novices, were taught the Rules of Facilitation and practiced the Communication Skills until a level of competency was achieved in the TIR workshop as indicated by the instructor.

The International Critical Incident Stress Foundation (ICISF) presents conferences at locations around the world. ICISF also sponsors courses utilizing crisis intervention techniques and strategies. In my opinion, incorporating the Rules of Facilitation and Communication Skills into the curriculum of courses that teach crisis intervention techniques would be beneficial for students of the subject. CISD students could then have the advantage that TIR students gain from this set of knowledge and skills. Of course, graduates of CISM training as well as TIR training have the will to help and of course they all get better and better with experience. The point here is that all CISD graduates would benefit from these specific aspects of TIR training.

ICISF ensures in each curriculum that continuous assessment take place during and immediately after any type of crisis intervention, whether it is 1:1, defusing or CISD. In addition, the training includes practice in crisis intervention techniques and group processes. However, not all students are familiar with the person centered approach. Some of the CISD facilitators are human services providers and are geared to the "fix-it" approach, rather than allowing the participant to determine the outcome on his/her own. TIR Rules of Facilitation and Communication Skills give the student the confidence that if the method is followed, the negative charge will be released. This makes it less likely that the facilitator will feel the urge to jump in and explain and interpret for the client, rather than just listening and sticking to the method in use.

All CISD facilitators seek the goal that in TIR terminology is called an *end point*. An *end point* can be defined as the optimum time to end any procedure, namely when a success has occurred. Indications appear. The client will feel and manifest relief from troubling emotions. (AMI/TIRA, 2006). Although CISD facilitators do not recognize *end points* per se, it is apparent to them that participants are "lightening up" once again by smiling, laughing and joking around. I have found the concept of an end point to be very useful in my work. This concept would help CISD facilitators to identify those individuals who have not discharged the negative charge and who might need further assistance. When this occurs after the CISD has culminated, the individual needing further intervention has not released all the material from the critical incident or from a former one. This is an indication that the CISD facilitator needs to spend time afterwards with the participant. Seasoned CISD facilitators perceive this readily, of course. Novice peer facilitators usually rely on the mental health professional on the team to identify who might need further follow-up. In severe incidents, such as drowning, burn victims, death of children or adolescents, there may be a need for many 1:1 interactions afterward. Applying the concept of *end points* is a very useful tool for CISD teams.

Peers, chaplains and mental health professionals who conduct CISD and other interventions that recognize proficiency and assist participants in releasing negative charges are naturally applying the principles of TIR Rules of Facilitation and Communication Skills. They have the intuitive ability to recognize what is indicated in each step and routinely experience successful debriefings. Specific training in these skills speeds the process of a person moving from novice to fully effective practitioner. One idea would be for this skill set to be included in CISD training. Another idea would be for people wishing to be crisis responders (or other professionals who meet trauma head-on) to take both CISD and TIR training.

Bibliography

AMI/TIRA. (2006). *Traumatic Incident Reduction Workshop Manual, 5th Ed.* Ann Arbor, MI: AMI Press.

Caplan, G. (1961). *An Approach to Community Mental Health.* New York: Grine and Stratton.

Caplan, G. (1964. *Principles of Preventive Psychiatry.* New York: Basis Books.

Everly, G.S., Jr. & Mitchell, J.T. (1999) Critical Incident Stress Management (CISM): A New Era and Standard of Care in Crisis Intervention. Ellicott City, MD: Chevron.

Flannery, R.B., Jr. (1998). *The Assaulted Staff Action Program.* Ellicott City, MD: Chevron.

Mitchell, J.T. & Everly, G.S., Jr. (2001) *Critical Incident Stress Debriefing: An Operations Manual for CISD.* Third Edition. Ellicott City, MD: Chevron.

Mitchell, J.T. (2004). Characteristics of Successful Early Intervention Programs. *International Journal of Emergency Mental Health*, Vol. 6, No.4, pp.175-184; Chevron.

Mitchell, J.T., Everly, G.S., Jr., Clark, D.W, (2006). *Strategic Response to Crisis Student Manual.* Ellicott City, MD: International Critical Incident Stress Foundation.

	CISD and TIR Training:
4	**Strange Bedfellows or Soulmates?**
	By Carlos Velazquez–Garcia
	Lic. Clinical Psychologist, CT

About the Author

Carlos Velazquez-Garcia is a licensed clinical psychologist in private practice in Puerto Rico. He trained both at Universidad de Puerto Rico and the Doctoral Clinical Psychology Program at NYU (ABD). He is a certified traumatologist and has the designation of Master traumatologist from the International Institute of Traumatology formerly at Florida State University. Carlos is the executive director of The Traumatology Center for Puerto Rico, a licensed site by The Academy of Traumatology, founded and presided over by Dr. Charles Figley. This center trains mental health professionals in CISD, TIR, EMDR and Cognitive Behavioral Therapy (CBT) with an international faculty.

Introduction

An active ingredient in most trauma therapies is the re-exposure of the victim to the traumatic event. One way that this is accomplished is by allowing the victim the opportunity to develop the oral narrative of the critical incident or traumatic event.

Critical Incident Stress Debriefing (CISD) and Traumatic Incident Reduction (TIR) both have the oral narrative of the critical event as an essential component of their protocol. I believe that the TIR emphasis on the Rules of Facilitation and the Management of Communication in its interventions can inform and significantly enhance the CISD intervention and its benefits. In this belief, I am very much in agreement with Jill Boyd (see Chapter 3).

CISD is one small group technique fundamental in the Critical Incident Stress Management Program developed by Mitchell and Everly (1998) as part of crisis intervention. A CISD session involves seven steps: Introduction, Facts, Thoughts, Reaction, Symptoms, Teaching and Re-entry. Each member of the group is given opportunity to share the facts, thoughts, and reactions of the critical event and is also educated about PTSD symptoms, resources available for aftercare and the last part is for achieving closure for the debriefing session. CISD can be done on an individual basis too.

The theory from which *CISD* evolves is The Two-Factor Theory (Everly, 1995). Essentially, it states that after one interprets an event as a threat, two factors emerge: 1) the physiological, which is the body's response to "fight or flee" from the threat; 2) the psychological factor, which is the mind's work trying to make sense of the experience that has shaken or shattered one's assumptions about the world (i.e. "no longer safe"), oneself (i.e. "I'm really a coward"), others ("people don't care", "all are mad").

D. Michenbaum (1993) has argued that "individuals tend to engage in internal and external dialogues that *fabricate meaning* (my emphasis) when the automaticity of their acts and scripted routines is interrupted and when readjustment is required" (p.708). This is so more when exposure to markedly stressful events calls for readjustment. Furthermore, Michenbaum, quoting Epstein (1990), observes, "threatening events invalidate at a deep experiential level the most fundamental beliefs in a personal theory of reality...[moreover], recovery is contingent upon building a new assumptive world that can assimilate the victimization experience in an adaptive manner" (p.80).

The world view that will remain after the meaning-making process evolves (Factor 2) will determine how affect, feelings, behavior, and sensations are normalized and/or integrated. This also depends on the cognitions that are accepted, whether erroneous or realistic. In the best case scenario the meaning-making process will yield cognitions and a world view that is adaptive. If the conclusion is that the world is not safe (generalization) then Factor 1, the physiological response, will remain in place and the person will/may develop maladaptive responses to deal with the physiological response that signals continued distress. With the continued presence of a heightened physiological state (Factor 1), the mind (Factor 2) will continue to try and deal better, find a better schema to assimilate the experience. Therefore the recurrence of memories, affects, etc. in PTSD can be interpreted as both a somatic and a mental attempt to "re-vision", "re-visit" the experience and the meanings attached to the original crisis or traumatic event, until it finds the best schema to make sense of the experience and sustain an adaptive world view.

Therefore, it follows that it is essential that people be given the opportunity to make explicit their experience regarding the critical event, that is, feelings, sensations, affects, behaviors, and their assumptions attached to these experiences; be they the ones that have been shattered (Janoff-Bulman, 1995) or the ones that remain intact. This will allow for the development of more adaptive schemas and responses. This will lead to the subsidence of the physiological and psychological factors that were activated.

Traumatic Incident Reduction (TIR) is an individual technique, more oriented to the post crisis period, that is, when trauma symptoms (and possibly a diagnosis of PTSD) are present (French and Harris, 1999).

In both techniques, **the oral narrative** of the critical incident is essential. TIR utilizes a protocol that requires iterations of the critical incident or traumatic event until an End Point is reached. An End Point is:

...the moment when 'indicators' appear
that make it clear that the client has visibly
relaxed and 'lightens up'. (p.17, French and
Harris, op. cit.)

Also the client's attention "comes out of the past into
the present (extroversion)" and "often the client has some
insight."

According to Dr. Charles Figley (1983):

"The trauma victim marks the move from victim to survivor by answering five survivor's questions with little or
no negative affect."

1. What happened?
2. Why did it happen?
3. Why did I act as I did at the time of the traumatic
   event?
4. Why she/he acted as she/he has since the traumatic event?
5. What will happen if the traumatic event happens
   again?"

French and Harris further state (pages 6-7):

"In essence, the victim makes sense of the traumatic
experience and by allowing it to fit with the self and the
model of the world, becomes stable and completes the integration process by assimilating and accommodating the
event into the schema."

Gerbode (1995) states that "for any trauma to remain
emotionally charged and unresolved, part or all of a traumatic incident must remain uninspected" (p. 436). The
event has been incompletely examined and therefore the
victim has been unable to make sense of it. The TIR procedures provide the opportunity to revisit the event until
the response is transformed."

Now it is clear that both CISD and TIR are intent on allowing the client to "re-inspect," "re-visit," "re-view" the critical experience in order to develop better schemas that make sense and allow for adaptive meanings to emerge. In this process, the most important aspect is the emerging **oral narrative of the incident** as the evolving construction and expression of the meaning.

TIR facilitates the client's full awareness of the experience of the traumatic event. This is accomplished via the management of communication and the Rules of Facilitation (see Appendix C). These two essential components of TIR training can very effectively become part of the "debriefer" facilitative tools.

Management of Communication in TIR

French and Harris state (p. 26):

"The skill required of a facilitator has nothing to do with his/her knowledge of the theory or technique of TIR. Rather it lies in expert managing of communication in the session while adhering strictly to the Rules of the Facilitation. These skills enable you to create a suitable and safe place in which viewing (of the critical event) can take place."

In order to fully revisit the traumatic event, it is imperative that the client's full attention be available to focus on the emotional, cognitive, iconic (visual memory), and echoic (physical sensation memory) elements of that event. Any mismanagement of communication on our part will cause the client's attention to be pulled outward, to us, rather than inward to the event (the experience), reducing the possibility of examining the event as fully as possible with all the elements of the experience. When this experience is made available, first sub-symbolically (internally) and then in oral language (symbolically), it will facilitate a deeper sense, meaning of/for the experience.

Bucci's (1995) work supports the importance of first attending inwardly to gather information that may have been encoded non-verbally, before giving it verbal expression, that is before giving the oral narrative of the traumatic experience. Bucci indicates that we have a multi-coding system of registering experience: symbolic and sub-symbolic. The symbolic includes verbal and non-verbal forms. The sub-symbolic modes all are nonverbal. Language is an example of a symbolic code. It is primarily a cortical process. Emotion is a sub-symbolic code, and is mainly in the limbic system. This corresponds to cortically processed experience via language, and sub-cortically in limbic-registered *experience.* Please note that there are other sub symbolic forms of registering experience: for example, visceral and motoric forms.

The client needs to make meaning of the traumatic experience. Evolving an oral narrative is a way of doing so. Inwardly focused attention on the memories and the affects, sensations, and behaviors that were registered symbolically *and* sub-symbolically adds an enormous amount of information that helps this process. As these affects, sensations, etc. are allowed to emerge, and bit by bit inform the evolving oral narrative of the event, it will be made "whole" or more integrated, with fewer elements dissociated or unavailable.

TIR: Communication and The Rules of Facilitation.

Wendy Coughlin, Ph.D. wrote in an unpublished paper: "TIR provides a paradigm for accessing traumatic material *through the client's associational pattern* (my emphasis) without directing the content."

TIR training maximizes the role of the facilitator in helping the client become aware of the experience via the deceptively simple Communication Skills and Rules of Facilitation (see Appendix C).

The goal of TIR is to allow the client to become aware of and process the traumatic experience, and provide an opportunity for the oral narrative to emerge and lead to meaning. The Rules of Facilitation are essential for achieving this goal.

The Rules of Facilitation proposed by TIR significantly provide for achievement of the goal of allowing the client to become aware and process their experience and provide the opportunity for the oral narrative to emerge as a meaning-making opportunity.

Note that rule #10 "Carry each viewing action to a success for the viewer" is a therapeutic goal which would not apply to a CISD session.

Some of the Rules of Facilitation are implicitly or even explicitly considered in CISD Training (Mitchell & Everly, 1988). TIR training more fully develops these skills and makes their rationale explicit.

Facilitating the debriefers' work: One way of maximizing the benefits of CISD sessions would be by enriching the training of the debriefers, as TIR does for its facilitators, through the management of communication. They would benefit from being exposed to the Communication Exercises and the utilization of the Rules of Facilitation (see Appendix C). This would certainly add to the CISD goal of allowing the participants to experience, as fully as possible, their role, reactions, etc. to the critical event.

Steven Gold (2000) comments:

"There are a number of reasons why we consider TIR preferable to other techniques with similar aims." I summarize them here: (1) There is empirical evidence that it is more effective than other exposure methods (Bisbey, 1995). (2) The client is clearly in charge of directing the exploratory and explanatory process. (3) It allows the client to arrive at his/her own understanding of the incident.

Gold concludes: "Consequently, TIR bolsters the client's sense of empowerment and promotes the capacity for self sufficiency that is integral to the contextual approach to treat Prolonged Child Abuse (PCA) survivors." (p. 220).

Summary: CISD is a crisis intervention technique that aims to provide processing of potentially traumatic experience before maladaptive responses arise and become entrenched to deal with both physiological and psychological reactions to the critical events.

TIR is a metapsychological technique that facilitates the processing of traumatic material in order to reduce its deleterious impact. Both agree on the essential reproduction of an emerging oral narrative that is a corrective/transforming meaning making opportunity.

TIR has developed crucial understanding and training by managing communication and the development of rules of practice that can surely inform and enrich CISD sessions as well as other similar techniques. My hope and goal is to make more explicit the rationale and importance of some elements of TIR training toward the goal of preventing and or alleviating the negative consequences of exposure to potentially or actually traumatic experiences.

Q&A with Carlos Velazquez–Garcia

Victor: How does CISD fit with the person-centered model as used in Metapsychology?

Carlos: Regarding CISD and the person oriented model:

1. CISD is person-oriented since the client is the ultimate authority over his experience. No interpretations are allowed by the facilitators or fellow participants. It is neither group therapy nor individual therapy in a group setting. It is an opportunity to share experience, thoughts, emotions, information, in a group of fellow witnesses to tragedy.

2. Participants do not have to talk if they don't want to. Nor they are forced to come to the debriefings.

3. Much like TIR, CISD is also directive. It provides structure and control, gives participants instructions and questions in adequate sequence and organizes and keeps track of the session progress. The facilitator in CISD also tries to handle communication smoothly.

Victor: CISD as done in a group setting instead of the one-on-one approach of TIR is a point of contrast. How is the element of being "safe to say anything" constructed in the group context?

Carlos: CISD is done in small groups of about 12 people. In the field, you might have groups of 18 people. Hopefully there would be one mental health worker and two trained peers leading the group. Safety comes from the assurance of confidentiality "what is said here remains here." It is specified that there will be no note taking by anyone, nor members of the press present. Only those who have witnessed the critical event participate in the group. All are invited to share; you don't have to if you do not desire to do so. By just being there you can gain from the others experience.

Victor: Is it true that most CISD is done in a time-limited treatment plan?

Carlos: It [CISD] is expected to last from 1.5 to 3 hours. It is not time-limited. You schedule the groups, one in the morning and one in the afternoon so that leaders do not become too "fatigued". It is far better to run different groups by different leaders, than several groups by the same leaders the same day.

Victor: In the trauma-treatment timeline, my assumption has always been that CISD is done much closer to the actual event (literally within in days or hours) whereas TIR requires the incident to be complete before it can be addressed with a client in a more stable condition. Is this the case?

Carlos: Defusings are shorter versions and less structured versions of debriefing that are done closer to the event (within 12 hours). **Debriefings**, CISD, are more structured and are done from 2 to 10 days of the event. I typically do debriefings about 3 weeks after trauma. My experience is that if it's too soon, the person is often unable to benefit.

Victor: I've often thought of CISD as a triage technique where those people identified with severe traumatic stress could be referred on to more comprehensive techniques like TIR. Can you comment on CISD as a screening for TIR?

Carlos: CISM, or Critical Incident Stress Management program, of which CISD is one component, includes an educational or informational component that incorporates or provides for the need of referral and even for follow up visits, i.e. by clergy if appropriate. Within the CISD session, there is one (educational) stage where people are familiarized with PTSD symptoms and related phenomena that might appear weeks after the event and are given information of mental health facilities that are prepared to assist them. Also they are alerted to possible more immediate needs, like suicidal potential in some of the participants. After the group ends, they are immediately assessed for risk and the emergency hospitalization proceeds as a matter of course. In the educational phase, people can be introduced to techniques like TIR and Facilitators in the area that they can contact as need arises.

Again, thank you for the opportunity to contribute in some way to your work in disseminating the effectiveness and possible applications of TIR Training.

Victor: Thank you, Carlos, for your observations.

References

Bucci, W. The Power of the Narrative: A Multiple Code Account, in J. W. Pennbaker *Emotions Disclosure and Health* APA, Washington, D. C. (ed. 1995)

Bisbey, L. B. *No Longer a Victim, A Treatment Outcome Study for Crime Victims with PTSD*.Doctoral dissertation, CSPS, 1995 – D.A.I., 5, 1692

Epstein, S. Natural Healing processes of the Mind. In D. Meichenbaum and M. Jaremko (eds) *Stress prevention and Management*. Plenum Press, 1983.

Everly, G. S. "An Integrative Two-Factor Model of Post-Traumatic Stress," Chapter 3, in G.S. Everly and J. M. Latig (Eds), *Psychotraumatology: Key Papers and Core Concepts in Post Traumatic Stress*, Plenum Press, New York 1995

Figley, C. R. *Catastrophes: An Overview of Family Reactions* (1983) in Figley & McCubbin (Eds) *Stress and the Family (Vol. II) Coping with Catastrophe*, Brunner/Mazel, 1983.

French, G. D. and Harris, C. J. *Traumatic Incident Reduction (TIR)* (1999), CRC Press, Florida, USA

Gerbode, F.A. *Beyond Psychology: An Introduction to Metapsychology (3rd Ed.)* (1995) IRM Press, Menlo Park, CA

Gold, S. *Not Trauma Alone*, (2000), Brunner/Routledge, Philadelphia, PA

Janoff-Bulman, R. (1995) Victims of Violence.Chapter 6 in G.S. Everly and J. M. Latig (Eds), *Psychotraumatology: Key Papers and Core Concepts in Post Traumatic Stress*, Plenum Press, NY 1995.

Meichenbaum, D.and Fitzpatrick,D (1993) A Constructivist Narrative Perspective on Stress and Coping: Stress Inoculation Applications. In Leo Goldberguer and Schlomo Breznitz(eds.) *Handbook of Stress , Theoretical and Clinical Aspects.* 1993, 2nd Ed.. The Free Press NY, NY.

Mitchell, I. T. and Everly, G. S. *Critical Incident Stress Management: The Basic Course Workbook* (2nd Edition) ICISF, Inc. (1998), Elliot City. MD, USA

Rogers, S. and Silver, S.M Is EMDR an Exposure Therapy? A Review of Trauma Protocols. *Journal of Clinical Psychology*, Vol 58 (1), p. 43-59 (2002)

Stickgold, R. EMDR: A Putative Neurobiological Mechanism of Action, *Journal of Clinical Psychology*, Vol. 58 (1), p. 61-75. 2002

CISM, TIR and Workplace Crime: A Conversation with Gerry Bock

Victor: How did you become involved with the Critical Incident Stress Management field and what training have you had?

Gerry: I first became involved as a child, witnessing the events going on in my own neighborhood and being a "go to person" for my peers, when traumatic events occurred. I have always felt quite comfortable in the midst of difficult circumstances and I had frequent encouragement from my peers to exercise and explore this gift. I believe that the roots of this ability may have come from the attitudes I developed in my upbringing in the Northwest Territories. In Inuvik, nobody locked their doors and people were highly dependent upon others in the community for survival. In the NWT, there was a very well developed sense of community, and when difficulty struck in any form, there were naturally occurring debriefing sessions in cohesive groups, not too different form what we currently call CISD interventions.

Later in life, our family moved to Alberta, and it seemed like peers and acquaintances, who were experiencing difficult family challenges or who were victims of troubling circumstances, would turn to me for assistance. I was there to help. I was involved in many traumatic and sometimes complex circumstances throughout my school years. In high school, I studied as much psychology as was offered at the time. My attitude in approaching most situations has always been, "If we can come together and mobilize resources as a community, we can manage to resolve almost anything."

It is no surprise then, that with my experiences and early success in assisting others, I ended up in a helping profession. In the early 1980s, I made the decision to get formal training. I first attended university courses in crisis counseling, then the Justice Institute of British Columbia where I studied about how trauma affects the workplace. I met Gerald French and Marian Volkman at an Association of Traumatic Stress Specialists (ATSS) conference and after being hooked into the phenomenal success and simplicity of Traumatic Incident Reduction, I began arranging for the TIR courses to be presented regularly in British Columbia. I am now certified as a Traumatic Stress Specialist with ATSS and am an active member of the trauma responder community.

Victor: I understand that you get called in frequently after a bank robbery. Walk me through a typical scenario. For example, a bank has just had a robbery incident. The teller had a gun waved in her face and shots were fired but nobody was hurt. Bring me through the whole series of activities you undertake.

Gerry: First of all, I make my phone call with my contact person and ask whether there is anyone I should be especially concerned about or who is observed to be "at risk." If there is, I might want to talk to that person on the phone while I'm en route to the intervention or in some manner be sure that that person is receiving attention and support. I will also gather as much information as possible prior to my arrival, so that I can conduct a preliminary assessment of who may be most at risk and what could be done for them. For a situation like the one you described, I'm probably being called in for an immediate defusing. That means I'll grab my briefcase, walk out the door, bringing phone numbers of clients I need to reschedule, and be on my way within a few minutes to the site where the incident took place. Chances are the bank will be closed for the balance of the day or at least for a few hours in these situations. This temporary closure allows the police to conduct a preliminary investigation and gather evidence, while also allowing for staff to regroup, mobilize emotional resources as needed and complete administrative procedures.

If I do talk on the phone with tellers or other bank employees, I will ask them how they are doing and what it is that they are most concerned about. Sometimes, they're most concerned about "getting out from under the desk." They're hiding, still freaked out, even though they may not be the one the gun was waved at. I say, "It's no problem, stay there as long as you like. Make yourself comfortable, I'll be there in about 20 minutes and we'll discuss it." Sometimes, it is the staff that were not directly involved who are the most affected, so, I will never know exactly what I am walking into; as trauma responders we all need to be well prepared and fluidly creative in our approach.

I will gather all of the information possible beforehand, make tentative assumptions and plans, walk in with hope, confidence and a lot of good tools, then get to work, often revising the plan depending on how the situation unfolds while I am on site. I have read that military battles are like this, in that the best laid plans often come apart in execution, and that the most flexible and creative strategies are the ones that turn the tide.

When I get on site, I will further assess the situation. In circumstance where some people may still not be recognizing that the danger has passed and are still in hiding mode, I might use the Applied Metapsychology technique that includes: "Tell me something it would be safe to do?" or "Touch and let go" on objects within easy reach. These techniques help to calm and orient the frightened person enough, allowing emergence from hiding and potentially doing some reintegration with peers in the group meeting.

Then I ask the contact person to assemble the staff and I will conduct a group defusing (within a few hours of an incident) or a debriefing. I would assure the staff and everybody present that the Employee Assistance Program and I are available to work with the group to bring about a return to calm and normal functioning. Sometimes a joke or two comes up about the length of time required to bring about normal functioning in the work place, such as having the trauma responder camp out at the branch for a few weeks. Humor can lighten up a serious situation. It is important to identify the goals of a trauma intervention early on and inform the staff what they can expect as an outcome from the meeting and my on-site intervention.

I then carry on with the defusing/debriefing, starting with the psycho-educational piece. Psycho-education covers what the common or typical reactions are to a traumatic event and discussions about what can be done to respond effectively to these reactions. We discuss what to do if insomnia strikes, what to discuss, and how to discuss the day's events with family and friends, and so on. Frequently during the early part of the peer meeting, discussions will arise about how the event was handled and what can be learned from it. We will also identify and discuss resilience: what characteristics do they have as the staff of that bank, what they are doing well as a community, what resources do they have, what do they need from each other, and so on.

After the group work, I'll meet one-on-one with anyone who wants (or may need) to do so, especially those who have been identified as potentially at risk. There will be some who I will specifically ask to meet with as a matter of routine. If it was a case of "gun waved in her face and shots fired," I would start with the employee who had the gun waved in her face and any person who was hiding under or behind the desk and was afraid to come out after the incident was over. I make sure that nobody who may be at risk goes home unaccompanied, and encourage staff to not be alone in the next 24 - 48 hours and to engage in some vigorous exercise at some point within the next 24 hours. In the circumstances you've described, I might have 2 or 3 other CISD trained counselors with me. I always request counselors who are trained in both CISD and TIR if they are available.

Victor: Does it ever involve working with customers?

Gerry: Sometimes, but rarely. It depends on the bank; anyone who was affected, I would follow-up with as a matter of routine regardless (though in some circumstances, the EFAP[1] counselor will follow up on my behalf). If there were customers in the bank, I would not necessarily contact them on my own initiative. I would first clear with the bank staff whether they would like the scope of the intervention to be expanded to customers (which they may desire, depending on the circumstances). Then I would ask the bank staff to contact persons who are not employees and ask if they would like to speak with a counselor. If a customer was very upset, the bank employee would typically ask if it would be OK for a counselor to call. In some cases, the customers may still be in the branch when I arrive and I have opportunity to interact with them and possibly do a short intervention with later follow up.

It is much more common to involve people who are not staff members (typically family members), in circumstances where there has been a sudden death of an employee. It is not generally advisable to invite non-employees to a group defusing or debriefing intervention, as these meetings need to be homogenous in nature, to allow peers to be able to share with each other in a safe space. Even the involvement of managers and administrators in a group meeting is typically a decision made on site by the lead counselor.

---

[1] The Employee & Family Assistance Program (EFAP) is an off-site, confidential, voluntary, short-term counseling service. It is different from other programs as it acts as a separate entity under a non-profit society concept.

Victor: What types of situations do you find yourself being called in for CISM?

Gerry: Critical Incident Stress Management (CISM) is a large category, with many counselors providing service for many different types of critical incidents. Statistically across Canada, many CISM interventions involve corporate downsizing and employee termination. Here on the west coast of British Columbia, I am called most frequently for resolving trauma related to bank robberies. I am also called out for traumatic grief, workplace accidents, and terminations (or layoffs) when employees may be at risk.

Victor: Where do you see TIR fitting in the scheme of CISM, which has a specific phase timeline related to the incident?

Gerry: Since I have learned about Applied Metapsychology and TIR, it has become the foundation for my entire clinical practice. I use TIR following a defusing, which is typically within a few hours of a traumatic event; or following a debriefing, which can be a few days to a few weeks after a critical incident.

During the more formal group sessions, I will observe who may be at risk, or who might benefit from TIR or Metapsychology techniques. I will typically make a mental list of these individuals, starting with the ones who appear to be the most affected; I will connect with them briefly one to one, and assess their level of functioning and state of mind following the group meeting. I will then arrange one to one sessions as appropriate, and use TIR or Metapsychology tools to resolve the impact of the traumatic stressors.

I have developed a whole new procedure that incorporates what I have found most useful to the process. My adapted procedure is as follows:

1. On site assessment and group meeting as per developed protocols—Observe and identify those individuals who may be at risk for ongoing, acute impact and arrange to meet with them one to one following the group meeting. Typically, I will have asked the contact person to arrange a private room for this purpose ahead of time.

2. During the one to one session, I begin with providing more in-depth psycho-educational information about PTSD and common reactions to traumatic events. I have an illustrated diagram about how traumatic (emotional) energy is created and what happens to it following an event. I continue to observe and assess responses during this phase, as well as identifying trigger areas. This way, I can determine which of the symptoms presented may be of concern, or of interest to the client. The potential impact of either resolving or leaving these issues also becomes clear.

3. Developing an impromptu treatment plan on the spot is the next step, using tools from the TIR workshops. Generally, the bulk of the resolution is brought about through the use of Basic TIR to an end point.

4. I usually then use a form of Future TIR (from the TIR Expanded Applications workshop) to consolidate the gains made in the session by first exploring the impact of having resolved the issues at hand, then checking for the development of potential future impacts, should a similar incident (or something related to the current incident) occur in the future. For example, using the impact of a bank robbery, I may run Future TIR on scenarios such as:
   a. Returning home after work and seeing the face of the robber in traffic or while out in public.

     b. Returning to work for the next scheduled shift (often the next day). Returning to work next week, next month, or in one year from today.

     c. Being robbed again in the next day, the next week, the next month, or the next year(s).

5. Typically I would then check all flows[2] on the original incident.

6. The entire process, usually fresh in the mind of the viewer (client), brings the gratification of rapid relief, typically in 20 – 50 minutes, though it can be as long as 90 – 120 minutes.

Victor: Given that CISM has a sort of built-in triage aspect, how do you determine which people get which type of follow-ups?

Gerry: Follow-up is done, if possible, on site with each person who displays symptoms of impact from the incident. The way that I think of impact is that if you were there, it has impacted you and left you with some type of emotional charge. What I am looking for is the following:

     a. What level of emotional charge does this person have?

     b. What have they done with the emotional charge? Have they repressed, suppressed, dismissed, ignored or resolved the impact of the incident? If they have resolved it, no further action is required on my part. If any of the other responses are in place, it is a question of facilitating the eventual resolution of the impact through psycho-education; a one-on-one session there and then if appropriate; referral; or allowing the individual to seek assistance, if desired, at a later time and place.

---

[2] See p. 139 for an explanation of *flows* in Applied Metapsychology.

Sometimes, if there are unresolved concerns, I will ask a client I have met with one to one for permission to follow up by telephone. I also may ask the employer to contact employees who may be at risk, or those who have chosen to opt out (or who could not be present) during a formal session for some reason or another. The employer would contact the individuals and ask if it would be acceptable for me to contact them by telephone, perhaps while I am still on site. My goal is always to leave a site or complete a case after having reached an end point for all employees. Although I am typically in and out within a few hours, sometimes I can be on site for two or three days, because of the large number of employees affected. Sometimes, I need to bring a second or even a third counselor with me, if there are a large number of people affected by a traumatic incident.

Of course, we all develop intuition and the ability to make sound clinical judgments and this improves with experience and training in CISM. I always try to get "tuned in" by putting myself into the mindset of the people I am dealing with and then paying close attention to what is being said (or not said). I know when I approach a situation that emotional energy (charge) has been created by the incident; I know it has to be dealt with and resolved in some form. I am really assessing how much charge has been developed and whether it is being resolved, and approach people with that in mind, looking to solve the mystery of how they are dealing with the impact of the incident.

Victor: You mentioned clients who may not be aware of the impact... Is there an aspect of people going into denial?

Gerry: With men, I frequently get a response like "I'm not affected," or "I'm fine." Men in particular may refuse to talk to me or they sit down and say, "I'm fine, you know," as an opening sentence, even from one who was the most directly involved in the incident.

Victor: So that's a warning flag, if they seem completely blasé... or unresponsive?

Gerry: Right, because the energy developed by a traumatic incident has to go somewhere. Someone sits down and says "I'm fine." I say "OK, let's just check it." I ask a series of questions like, "How are you going to feel coming to work tomorrow?" I also check on the flows as well:

- How does standing next to the teller who was robbed feel?
- How does having lunch with [branch personnel] feel?
- How does your family feel when you tell them about it?

We might use Subjective Units of Distress (SUDs) or something less formal to measure the actual impact. Sometimes, the employee is not aware of how the incident has affected him or her and I need to ask these sorts of "let's check" questions to bring the emotional charge into their awareness. Typically, clients are appreciative that I have been thorough in checking this out with them when they become aware of how the incident has affected them. This is especially true when the "awareness of impact" becomes "resolution of impact" and they leave a session feeling much better.

Victor: How soon can you deliver TIR after a workplace incident?

Gerry: I have delivered TIR highly successfully after only 30 minutes following an incident, though often it is a few hours at the earliest.

Victor: Does your observation or experience differ from CISM experts in this regard?

Gerry: There are a lot of different opinions from the experts about how soon to deliver an intervention or whether to have any intervention at all.

Based on my own experience, it is always best to have an intervention of some type (even a short or limited one) as soon as possible, so that the people impacted can have a greater sense of direction and feel connected to assistance and develop a plan for resolution. Typically, the worst for someone who has been impacted is the sinking feeling that the trauma has made them into "helpless victims". I believe strongly in a message of hope through collaboration and skilled resolution to an end point.

Victor: Are there TIR facilitator skills that improve your effectiveness as a CISM provider?

Gerry: Yes, absolutely! Having been formally trained in the traditional forms of debriefing first, and then experiencing what TIR and Metapsychology could do with a traumatic incident, opened up a whole new dimension of thinking about trauma and what is required to resolve it successfully.

As a clinical counselor, with a master's level of training and over 15 years of professional experience in the field, I believe I had become very focused on specific and favorite modalities, using very specific skills. I was very humbled to learn that there was a different, and potentially more efficient, and much more effective way to resolve trauma. Perhaps the most humbling was the realization that this new way of resolving trauma was not at all dependent upon my own knowledge and theories. In my experience, TIR is highly dependent upon my skills and ability in building rapport early and quickly and then empowering the client to come to an end point (resolution) on their own terms.

After reading the book entitled *Traumatic Incident Reduction* by French & Harris, I knew that I had to learn this modality as soon as it could be reasonably arranged. I was not disappointed.

In a CISM situation, a counselor needs to be well tuned to what is going on with clients who may not be aware of the impact; as a TIR facilitator, the counselor needs to be able to listen and respond quickly, inspiring confidence and competence. I now use the skills I have gained from my TIR training in every clinical situation that I am involved with. The following are some of the most important skills I have learned:

The Communication Exercises taught in the TIR Workshop are phenomenal for any type of relationship that has been fractured or traumatized. I also find these to be a great benefit for being an effective counselor in virtually any situation. I am reminded frequently of how important this is, when I hear my own assumptions being shattered by the reality of what is really going on in the mind of a client. The ability to listen with intention, using the communication exercise skills and the rapport building tools have really increased my effectiveness as a counselor in CISM and other circumstances quite dramatically.

The Rules of Facilitation (see Appendix C) are incredibly powerful for making a client feel empowered, to find hope, and to identify resilience in the face of seemingly overwhelming circumstances. The personal hope for a better future comes from within, and the Rules of Facilitation create a space for this to arise. This is obviously different from creating years of dependency on a well-meaning service provider or agency, which sometimes happens. These Rules of Facilitation also cut the compassion fatigue factor to a much less significant concern.

The structure of the Metapsychology tools and TIR are easy to learn and use effectively. This helps to be able to adapt in CISM sessions quickly, easily and on the spot. The structure of these tools, once learned, rarely leaves a counselor feeling stuck. This has expanded the range of clients and issues that I am able to deal with, effectively and efficiently.

Victor: What insights have you had as a CISM provider in regard to how different people experience the same incident?

Gerry: The biggest insight I have gained is that there are no standard rules as to how clients will process an event. Each client needs to be provided the opportunity to process in a way that makes sense to him or her, for rapid and permanent resolution. Counselors need to be facilitators of clients' healing, not "experts". This is a humbling experience because the client is really working through it alone. It's not so much what you say that makes the difference; rather it comes about through the safe healing space you provide. Following the structure laid out in TIR and Metapsychology yields rapid and lasting results.

Victor: Which part of your work in these situations do you see as having the biggest impact on resilience of the client (in terms of future incidents?)

Gerry: For clients, knowing that they have faced and successfully resolved a traumatic situation allows them the resiliency and the courage to be prepared internally for whatever may come next. Once they know they can get through big or frightening traumatic situations, everyday life is less of a challenge and more of a joy. Anxiety about future events is significantly lessened when current and past traumas are resolved. The use of Future TIR can be a big factor in consolidating resiliency gains for the future wellbeing of any client.

Victor: Are traumatic incidents in the workplace different from other types of personal crime incidents? If so, how?

Gerry: Although either can have similar impacts on daily life and ability to function, in my experience crime incidents frequently feel to clients as if they are more "personal" in nature, and directed at a perceived personal vulnerability, inadequacy or failure. Personal crime incidents, especially if they occur at or near a place of residence, can also create difficulty in finding mental distance and/or the feeling of having a safe space at home. In a personal crime incident, the stakes are generally also higher, as it is typically you and your own wellbeing or family that is being threatened.

For example, I had a client who had his family home mildly vandalized in a random act by drunken teens. There was no attack or threat on his person. The police were called and the offenders arrested. He had lived with his family in this home for more than ten years, without any other similar incidents at all. Suddenly, he and his family no longer felt safe in this home and felt compelled to sell the house and move, motivated by a constant nagging feeling of being unsafe in the neighborhood.

When an incident happens in the workplace, there are many more options for restoring a safe place from which to heal. This is a place where you have defined start and end schedules, and routine activities. This is also a place that can be left behind at the end of the scheduled work day. Careers can be changed, workplace locations can be transferred and there is a greater sense of mental distance in a traumatic incident in the workplace. Also, the final outcome of any healing process is higher when the personal stakes involve a crime that occurs in someone's home or involves a family member.

Victor: Any success stories that you can share with us about TIR and workplace crime incidents?

Gerry: What stands out in my mind is that, following a debriefing process that included using TIR and Metapsychology tools, I've had bank tellers express compassionate or positive feelings toward the criminals who robbed them. This has happened more than once. The person gets to a level where the incident itself is resolved and then the teller's own natural compassion for people who were probably down-and-out comes through naturally. They often experience a sense of feeling sorry for the robber. A teller may say something like, "My goodness, isn't it sad that this person had to stoop so low as to rob us in order to get what they needed. When he is caught, I wonder it there is anything I can do for him?"

Victor: That is so totally unlike what is expected.

Gerry: Right, usually people are just angry, and their attitude is often, "Why me?" and "How dare they?" The whole point is that TIR does not dwell on that. As it is client-centered, TIR facilitates a counselor bringing out the best in the client. A teller will say things like, "And you know, the guy was so good-looking or young... Why would he throw his life away like that?"

Victor: Is there anything you can say about resilience in terms of someone being robbed a second time?

Gerry: I get called out a lot because employees ask for me, so I'm often going to the same bank 3 to 4 times (or more) per year. Someone who had been through the process with me before may want to achieve a similar result where experiencing a robbery became a positive experience for them instead of a negative one. To me, the desire to have a positive experience after a traumatic event is quite a resilient attitude!

Some banks are robbed every few weeks or months, it just happens that way. In some cases, the same bank has been robbed several times in the same week. Some tellers tell me they have been through 15 or 20 of these incidents. In Canada, we have a lot fewer guns around[3] and so a bank robbery might be just a "note passer" through the teller wicket. It's more frequent here that it is not an armed theft. It's very rare that someone actually gets hurt in a Canadian bank robbery. We would like the tellers to have a calm internal sense in such incidents so that they can respond to it without panicking during the theft. If they freeze up they may be viewed by the robber as unco-operative. With a goal of getting the robber outside the bank building as soon as possible, a teller needs to re-main as calm and focused as possible. Once the robber is outside the bank and the doors to the outside are locked, the robber cannot harm the employees or the customers. Often, a bank robbery will take less than 2 minutes in to-tal. If the teller is calm and treats it like a routine transaction, it will all be over very quickly and it less likely that something will go wrong or that someone will get hurt.

Victor: What things do you like best about CISM work?

Gerry: CISM work is always different, always changing and you never know what to expect when the call comes in. It is typically quite an adrenalin ride and a powerful feeling when you have brought successful healing to a group of clients. There is nothing like it in the world of clinical counseling that I have ever come across.

Victor: What things do you like best about TIR?

Gerry: Before TIR, I enjoyed CISM, though I was all too often "bringing it home." Without the use of the TIR tools, I often felt compassion fatigue and was limited in how

---

[3] The 1995 Firearms Act makes casual ownership of handguns ex-tremely difficult. Despite this fact, an RCMP study showed 22% of Canadian households own a shotgun or rifle. Additionally, 1 out of 6 gun owners in British Columbia have a handgun.

many cases I could deal with effectively during a specific time period. I often felt as if I wanted to be able to offer better conclusions and more effective resolution closure to clients. The way I see it, in a standard CISM debriefing or defusing, you are able to jump start the healing process and get colleagues coming together in a more positive direction. There is also a lot that can go terribly or horribly wrong during or following a critical incident session and this can be quite overwhelming for both counselor and clients.

So, what can a counselor do with that absolutely overwhelming sense of compassion that keeps bobbing up to the surface in CISM sessions, in spite of our best efforts to keep it in check? In the face of (sometimes very extreme) human pain and suffering, what do you think you may be able to do with your own feelings? Without TIR, we have to fall back on what has been prescribed as standard protocols. This typically means that the counselor gets the process kick started and refers those who are in need to another counselor or agency.

To me, this had always felt very unsatisfying. I am already on site, I have already established a good rapport with these clients and now I am to refer them on?

Now enter Metapsychology tools and TIR training. The formal defusing or debriefing session itself facilitates empowerment, so that clients are able to resolve much of the difficulties right there. It is a whole different approach. I am no longer there just to start the process, I am there to begin, run through and complete the entire event, right to an end point in most cases. What cannot resolved in the initial intervention can be resolved on site afterward, typically with a minimal amount of additional effort and resources.

What is not to thoroughly love and enjoy about learning and utilizing Metapsychology and TIR? I have the rewards of feeling really great about the work that I am facilitating, because the results are there.

Victor: Do you see value in having CISM providers who are trained in TIR and vice-versa?

Gerry: Yes of course! In my opinion, CISM providers who want to consistently resolve incidents instead of just jumpstarting the healing process need TIR training to achieve this. Counselors trained in TIR who desire to provide more effective services to groups will want to get trained in CISM procedures and protocols.

Both modalities can be enhanced by the skills and training that the other provides. CISM without TIR is missing the opportunities to complete the process. TIR without CISM training is missing the structure for working with and understanding the bigger process.

As I write this article, I am confident that there will be some experts (likely including my CISM instructor) who will disagree with my expressed outcomes and experiences. There may also be some TIR trained individuals (even trainers who routinely lead groups) who may feel that they are well enough trained in TIR and Metapsychology to do CISM without further training. My advice is to get training in both subjects, and see how your results can dramatically improve.

Comments and inquiries may be directed to the author via e-mail: gerry@bock.ca

[Ed. Note: The following article is reprinted from *Beyond Trauma: Conversations on Traumatic Incident Reduction, 2nd Ed.* (2005), also from Loving Healing Press.]

To learn more about the Green Cross Projects and what they do, please skip ahead to p. 105

Victor: Tell me about your professional background.

Karen: I went to school at the University of Tennessee in Knoxville and received a BA in Academic Psychology. A few years later I went on to Oklahoma and worked for People Inc., a community-based social service organization that provides services for Developmentally Disabled individuals. During my employment there, I was appointed coordinator of a program called the Oklahoma Children's Initiative. It was a program of several services including in-home counseling for at-risk youth or those reunifying with their families after being in State custody. The program incorporated three additional service agencies in seven counties in eastern Oklahoma. The job required me to supervise Master's level people, which I felt increasingly unqualified to do, so in 1996 I returned to Tennessee and earned a Masters in Social Work. I'm now certified and working toward licensure.

Victor: How did you become involved with the Green Cross Projects?

Karen: I was in Oklahoma at the time of the bombing and was supposed to be in the building on the day after it happened. The CEO of the organization I worked for then was affiliated with the Oklahoma Association of Youth Services. OAYS sponsored the Green Cross to provide

training in Oklahoma City for [traumatologist] responders
and people who were interested in becoming responders.
[Ed. Note: responders are the first people on the scene to
help.] These responders would deal with situations like
the Oklahoma City bombing, natural or man-made traumatic incidents. He contacted Dr. Figley and they brought
Green Cross to Oklahoma City and did a series of train-
ings.

Victor: So the Green Cross Projects got started right
after the Oklahoma City bombing?

Karen: Yes.

Victor: I've got kind of a fragmented view of the organization. Is the major outcome of GCP the yearly
conferences?

Karen: After 9/11, GCP progressed into redevelopment
mode to incorporate lessons learned during the New York
deployment. The mission hasn't changed. It is to provide
consultation, information and education and to be able to
provide trained traumatologists to respond to communities in need.

Victor: Is the focus on CISD?

Karen: To a certain extent, yes. The focus of the GCP is
on making traumatologists and their specialized tools
readily available in communities where they are needed.

Victor: For people who are not familiar with debriefing,
how would it look to an observer?

Karen: It looks like a support group where everyone
gets to talk about what they experienced and what they
think and feel about it. First of all you give group members some information about the process of the group,
setting ground rules for confidentiality and providing information about the stress reaction, symptoms they might
encounter, and possible coping skills. It is important to

normalize common reactions. Then you facilitate a group discussion by asking a series of questions designed to provoke emotional and cognitive responses to help people stabilize their reactions. Finally, you encourage group members to utilize private and community resources to meet additional treatment needs as appropriate.

Victor: Do you think TIR fits in well with the critical incident debriefing model?

Karen: Yes, I do. Yet the CISM techniques are designed to be utilized at different stages in the assimilation of the traumatic incident. In order to avoid iatrogenic effects, it is inappropriate to begin debriefing in the initial response during the acute phase. The psycho-education process can get in the way when people are alternating between avoidant and intrusive thought patterns[1].

Debriefing is designed to help people through the initial stages of the trauma. Debriefing works well, if not to prevent the development of PTSD, then at least to assist in the assimilation process during the acute phase. Unlike Debriefing, TIR is designed as a treatment methodology.

Victor: What was the impact of Green Cross Projects on the community in Manhattan after 9/11?

Karen: The first team arrived on 9/16. Response teams of approximately 14 traumatologists and compassion fatigue specialists were arranged in weekly rotations for 4 weeks. Several of us stayed behind to provide continuity. I think there were about 39 people altogether in weeklong shifts. I was there for almost 3 weeks of the 4 weeks' total.

We began the first day at our worksite, debriefing groups of up to 20 people. That was only the first day or

---

[1] "Why Does Critical Incident Stress Management Not Work?" by Bryan Bledsoe, posted on www.ParamedicInfo.CA.

two and the groups got smaller as we went along. I'm un-
sure of the total number of people we saw. I think we each
talked to close to 100 people in the first three days.

After about three weeks, we began to notice obvious
signs of healing. There were more conversations being
held in the halls and the elevators, more smiles, more
people returning to work on a daily basis. As far as impact
for those we served, only they can attest to that.

Victor: That's a remarkable commitment for people to
drop everything and go out there!

Karen: Yes, the response was awesome. I was ready to
go on 9/11. It doesn't happen that fast, you have to have
the logistical arrangements worked out.

It was really interesting to see the outpouring of assistance. Most team members got to New York on donated
private planes. Pilots with Air LifeLine also donated flights
to get some team members home after their rotation was
finished.

Victor: So you had relationships set up in advance?

Karen: And some just seemed to happen as we needed
them.

Victor: Were the people you saw emergency responders or survivors of 9/11?

Karen: Mainly we worked with witnesses; survivors;
and families, friends, or co-workers of those who were
lost. Some team members did report working with responders when off-duty at our designated work site.
That's a different process altogether, because when they're
coming off the site, for example firefighters, they'd come
off a shift and then a few hours later they're going right
back. They can't afford to get caught up in the emotion
that will interfere with the job they have to do. They don't
usually have the luxury of doing any sort of debriefing un-

til they're finished and they're not going back into the site again.

Victor: Were there unique challenges such as confusion over whether people were missing or dead?

Karen: By 9/16 there were still a lot questions. There was a lot of dissonance about the loss, with people going through the grieving process starting with disbelief or denial. We found a lot of people being stuck at various stages; there seemed to be no way of understanding and preparing for the suddenness of the loss.

Victor: Did you have an opportunity to use TIR when you were there?

Karen: Not really. We did do some debriefings, and utilized some other techniques that help during the acute phase. I utilized some of the TIR training, many of the Rules of Facilitation (see Appendix C) and ideas about communication. We did do debriefing and some work borrowing significant aspects of TIR. That was during the later part of my time there. The process was more modified than going through actual steps, because we didn't have that kind of time. As time went on, it became more difficult to work with individuals for any length of time due to reinstatement of their job duties and expectations.

Victor: Is there kind of a triage aspect to it, where you refer people?

Karen: Absolutely, that was a very large part of it. When you're dealing with trauma in the acute phase, you don't try to fix it. You assess, and let them know what's out there. You do what you can so that if someone is going to have continued problems with it, they'll know to get additional help.

We were actually assigned to one organization, a union in New York that did have an Employee Assistance Program (EAP) set up. So we got the people that needed additional counseling or treatment in touch with their EAP.

Victor: Is the idea with debriefing and the initial stages to get as many people exposed as possible to understanding the effects of trauma?

Karen: Yes, that was our initial aim. We also did debriefing training for potential responders in the area. We set up a Green Cross Projects chapter in the area and trained local counselors and therapists in response and compassion fatigue.

Victor: I was thinking compassion fatigue would be an important component there.

Karen: Especially, yes. During a Green Cross response to any emergency or disaster situation, we take compassion fatigue specialists with us or organize to have compassion fatigue specialists readily available. I see that as a very big component of what GCP is about.

[Ed. Note: Although compassion fatigue is certainly a factor for first responders on the scene of a disaster, whether natural or man-made, it is virtually unknown to practitioners of TIR for two reasons. One is that the traumatic event is over by the time you are employing TIR. The other is that the entire protocol supporting the use of TIR allows both client and practitioner to attain closure on each piece of work as they proceed. This is supported by the principle that each session is taken to an end point.]

Victor: In our terms, you'd say that you can't really do TIR until the incident is over. Many of the firefighters eventually stayed at ground zero for weeks and weeks.

Karen: The firefighters didn't want to leave the site. And yes, TIR is designed for use with past trauma, not necessarily the acute trauma reaction where most people have difficulty with concentration or distraction.

I was able to use some of the concepts of the TIR process with some people; some of the ideas from Unblocking and flow questions. [Ed note: She is referring here to looking at the various directions or "flows" of action: another causing something to self; self to another; another to another; self to self.] It wasn't running a full session and we didn't have a complete end point. They were still in the middle of it; they hadn't begun to completely process it.

Victor: I remember that was very poignant, the firefighters refusing to go off duty.

Karen: Yes, and it was not just the firefighters. We often saw the rescue dogs coming back to the hotels to rest and then return for their next shift. We also saw new members of the Coast Guard taking their oath in the hotel lobby, preparing to join the search and rescue mission.

Victor: That kind of answers my question of how do you handle clients who aren't ready for TIR.

Karen: If they're really not ready to get into it, then you don't do TIR. You start where the client is, and you don't do anything that they are not willing and ready to do. At some point, you have to make a therapeutic judgment too: Is it going to do more harm to get into this? If you're not going to have time to fully address the incident, then don't start the TIR. Using some of the key questions in TIR is what I mean by using a modified session.

Victor: What were some of the lessons learned from 9/11 responding—did you modify how GCP would respond next time?

Karen: We learned a whole lot about organization and logistics. We have actual written protocols now on how to logistically handle a deployment. We actually use an incident command structure, patterned after what an emergency response team would use.

Victor: Have you used any of the other Applied Metapsychology techniques such as Unblocking?

Karen: I use Unblocking more often than TIR because I find it's easily adapted into a conventional counseling session. I especially use it with clients with whom I have an established therapeutic relationship who are having difficulty addressing an issue that they have identified for treatment. I also use the repetitive question theme with paradoxical questions, sometimes with positive results. I think the key is using the techniques with appropriate clients at the appropriate times.

Victor: One thing that's been fascinating to me talking to all the different people using TIR is how they create a zone of safety for the client. Do you have any specific approaches?

Karen: It all goes back to therapeutic alliance, and the question of how do you build a therapeutic alliance? I think basically it's just being real with the client, being a real person. Letting them start from their comfort zone and not saying "OK, this is what we're going to do today." I avoid having a set start kind of approach.

Victor: Really stepping into the client centered approach there?

Karen: Exactly.

The Green Cross Projects: Who, What, and How

Information below has been excerpted from the Green Cross Projects website.

Who Are We?

The Green Cross Projects (GCP) was initially organized to serve a need in Oklahoma City following the April 19, 1995 bombing of the Alfred P. Murrah Federal Building. In 2004, GCP merged with Green Cross Foundation and emerged as the Green Cross Assistance (GCA) program. We are an international, humanitarian assistance organization, non-profit corporation comprised of trained traumatologists and compassion fatigue service providers. Most are licensed mental health professionals, all are oriented to helping people in crisis following traumatic events. The web address is http://gcprojects.org/

What Do We Do?

The GCA responds to requests from individuals, organizations, and other entities following a traumatic event. The requests can include any or all of the following:

1. Crisis assistance and counseling: helping those in shock to get back on their feet and access their natural coping methods and resources.

2. Assessment and referral services: identifying who is recovering properly from the traumatic event, who is not, why they are not recovering and what additional or other services are needed when and by whom.

3. Orientation and Consultation to Management: educating management about the immediate, week-to-week, and long term consequences of traumatic events for individuals, work groups, families, and larger systems.

4. Training, Education, and Certification: pre-paring management, human resources, employee assistance professionals, and service providers with sufficient guidance and competence to first do no harm to the traumatized, and to help them recover.

5. Family Resource Management: designing and implementing programs for strengthening and pro-moting family wellness in the wake of traumatic events, with special attention to young children.

6. Long-term trauma counseling: helping those unable to recover quickly from the trauma by pro-viding individual and group trauma and grief counseling.

These services are provided over varying periods of time and performed initially by members of a deployment team. They are transported into the impacted area within hours after the request is made. They stay from between 3-6 weeks or until local Green Cross Project members can relieve them.

How Do We Help?

The Mission of any deployment is to transform "vic-tims" into "survivors". Immediately following a traumatic event, victims attempt to address five fundamental ques-tions:

1. What happened to me (my family, my company, my neighborhood, my city, my country)? This is charac-terized by shock, disbelief, disorientation, confusion.

2. Why did it happen to me (us)? This is characterized by fear in addition to the above feelings.

3. Why did I (we) do what I did during and right after this disaster? This is characterized by guilt and

feelings of inadequacy in addition to all the above feelings.

4. Why have I (we) acted as I have (we have) since the disaster? This is characterized by confusion about their own sanity, worry that they will never recover, and all the other feelings noted above.

5. Will I (we) be able to cope if this disaster happens again?

Service Provision: Organized Assistance

Prior to and throughout the deployment, the GCA works with the host or client to clarify the mission of the deployment and specify measurable and attainable goals. Typically the services are provided in waves:

- Wave I (Days 1-10 following the disaster): Crisis stabilization, contacting local GCP members to establish a chapter for continuity of care.

- Wave II (Days 5-15): Stress management, social support, orientation of management.

- Wave III (Days 10-20): All of the above plus training, assessment and referral, and family resource development.

- Wave IV (Days 15-40): All of the above reactions plus grief and loss consultation and counseling.

In addition to providing services through the host, the GCA works with local providers for the purpose of continuity of care. By Wave IV the local providers outnumber of outside providers.

Entire article copyright © 2006 Green Cross Projects.

Appendix **A**	# FAQ for Practitioners ## Interested in Using ## TIR & Related Techniques

Contents:

1. What is TIR?

TIR is a brief, one-on-one, non-hypnotic, person-centered, simple and highly structured method for permanently eliminating the negative effects of past traumas. It involves repeated viewing of a traumatic memory under conditions designed to enhance safety and minimize distractions. The client does the most important work in the session; the therapist or counselor offers no interpretations or negative or positive evaluations, but only gives appropriate instructions to the client to have him view a traumatic incident thoroughly from beginning to end. Hence, we use the term "viewer" to describe the client and "facilitator" to describe the person who is helping the client through the procedure by keeping the structure of the session intact and giving the viewer something definite to do at all times. The facilitator's activity is confined simply to giving a series of set instructions to the viewer; there is no advice, interpretations, evaluations, or reassurances.

In what we call Basic TIR, which addresses known incidents, the viewer locates a specific trauma to be worked on—one with a specific, finite duration. This incident is treated like a "videotape". First, the viewer "rewinds" it to the beginning, then "plays" it through to the end—without talking about it while doing the viewing. *After* the viewing, the facilitator then asks what happened, and the viewer can then describe the event or the internal reactions to going through it.

After the completion of one viewing (and one description), the facilitator has the viewer "rewind the videotape" to the beginning and run through it again in the same fashion. The facilitator does not prescribe the degree of detail or content the viewer is to get on each run-through. The viewer will view as much as is relatively comfortable to view. After several run-throughs, most viewers will be able to contact the emotion and uncomfortable details in terms of the strengths of the emotion more thoroughly.

Typically, the viewer will reach an emotional peak after a few run-throughs and then, on successive run-throughs, the amount of negative emotion will diminish, until the viewer reaches a point of having no negative emotion about the incident. Instead, the person becomes rather thoughtful and contemplative, and usually comes up with one or more insights concerning the trauma, life, or the viewer's self. There is a display of positive emotion, often smiling or laughing, but at least manifesting calm and serenity. At this point, the viewer has reached an "end point" and the facilitator stops the TIR procedure.

In Thematic TIR, a specific feeling called a "theme" is used to discharge a sequence of related traumatic incidents.

A TIR session is not ended until the viewer reaches an end point and feels good. This may take anywhere from a few minutes to 3-4 hours. Average session time for a new viewer is about 90 minutes. Average total session hours to eliminate PTSD symptoms is 15 - 20 hours.

2. What is TIR useful for?

It is highly effective in eliminating the negative effects of past traumatic incidents. It is especially useful when:

a. Where a person feels affected by a specific trauma or set of traumas, whether a formal diagnosis of "PTSD" has been applied.

b. A person reacts inappropriately or overreacts in certain situations, and it is thought some past trauma might have something to do with it.

c. A person experiences unaccountable or inappropriate negative emotions, either chronically or in response to certain experiential triggers.

3. How long has TIR been in use?

TIR has been in use since 1984 in something similar to its current form. It has undergone minor modifications over the years, mostly in the interests of greater simplicity and teachability.

4. What is the anticipated outcome of TIR?

In the great majority of cases, TIR correctly applied results in the complete and permanent elimination of most PTSD symptomatology. It also provides valuable insights, which the viewer arrives at quite spontaneously, without any prompting from the facilitator and hence can "own" in their entirety.

By providing a means for completely confronting a painful incident, TIR can and does deliver the mastery of the situation that would be experienced by a person who had been able to fully confront the trauma at the time it occurred.

5. What are the contraindications and risks of TIR?

TIR is contraindicated for use with clients who:

   a. Are psychotic or nearly so. TIR is most definitely an exposure or uncovering technique and hence is not appropriate for such clients.

   b. Are *currently* abusing drugs or alcohol. Clients should avoid taking painkillers, sleeping pills, tranquilizers or drugs that may impair their physical or mental abilities for at least 24 hours prior to a viewing session. Some substances require a longer abstinence before viewing can take place.

   c. Are not making a self-determined choice to do TIR. For TIR to work, the client has to want to do it. If the client is there under duress (e.g., on court order) or trying to please someone, TIR will not work. It may be possible, however, to explain to a reluctant client what TIR is. The client must be motivated to do the work before starting.

d. Are in life situations that are too painful or threatening to permit them to concentrate on anything else. If the client is afraid of being murdered or engaged in violent fighting with his spouse, for instance, such issues/situations would have to be addressed first by consultation to develop a plan to handle the current life situation before the client will be ready to do TIR.

e. Have no interest in or attention on past traumas. A general rule is to follow the interest of the client. The larger subject of Applied Metapsychology includes a considerable array of techniques that help bring greater order and certainty to the viewer's mental environment.

Since the TIR technique is completely person-centered and non-forceful, clients will simply discontinue the procedure to protect themselves if they are getting in too deeply. Hence, there are no negative effects from properly facilitated TIR. If the facilitator were to try to *force* the client to run an incident, TIR could cause a considerable (though temporary) upset. But one of the cardinal Rules of Facilitation (see Appendix C) is never to force the client and always to follow the client's interest. Since we follow the client's interest at all times, we don't encounter resistance. If the client resists, we consider that we are not addressing the material the client should be looking at, at present.

6. What are the historical antecedents of TIR?

TIR grew mainly out of the work of Carl Rogers and Sigmund Freud. In *Two Short Accounts of Psycho-*

Analysis, Freud describes a method to resolve sequences of similar traumas:

> "What left the symptom behind was not always a *single* experience. On the contrary, the result was usually brought about by the convergence of several traumas, and often by the repetition of a great number of similar ones. Thus it was necessary to reproduce the whole chain of pathogenic memories in chronological order, or rather in reversed order, the latest ones first and the earliest ones last; and it was quite impossible to jump over the later traumas in order to get back more quickly to the first, which was often the most potent one."

Freud later abandoned this technique in favor of free-association. It seems likely that (in retrospect) the reason it didn't work well was the degree of interference the analyst introduced by interpretations and by forcing the analysand [client] in various ways, and the lack of a systematic, repetitive approach to achieving the desired anamnesis.

The work of Carl Rogers was invaluable in providing rules – such as a proscription against interpretations and evaluations – and an overall viewpoint of respect for the authority of the client, both of which we use to help create a safe environment for running TIR.

Although Rogers first described his work as "non-directive" and later as "person-centered", it seems obvious that "non-directive" doesn't mean the same thing as "person-centered". "Person-centered" describes the attitude of respect for the superior authority of the client and the concomitant rules for not stepping on the client's reality. "Non-directive" means the client gives structure to the session. These two are actually separate dimensions (see

Fig. 1). For instance, classical, free-associative psycho-analysis is non-directive, but not person-centered. Cognitive and behavioral therapies are non-person-centered (because the therapist disputes the reality of the client) [Ed. Note: that only applies to RET/REBT, not to other CBT.] and directive (the therapist determines the agenda). Rogers is non-directive and person-centered. TIR falls into the fourth category: person-centered *and* direc-tive, as the TIR facilitator provides structure for the client to be able to do the work of the session.

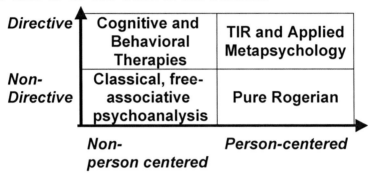

Directive	Cognitive and Behavioral Therapies	TIR and Applied Metapsychology
Non-Directive	Classical, free-associative psychoanalysis	Pure Rogerian

Non-person centered   *Person-centered*

Fig. A–1: Dimensions of Directive and Person–Centeredness

7. How and why does TIR work?

Freud based his work on the theory that in order to re-cover from past traumas, it is necessary to achieve a full anamnesis (recovery of lost memory). He never adequately explained *why* anamnesis was necessary; however let's consider a person centered explanation.

A trauma, by definition, is an incident that is so pain-ful, emotionally or physically, that one tends to flinch away from it, not to let oneself be aware of it, or, in Freud's terms, to repress it. It is the *flinch* and not the ob-jective content of the incident that makes it a trauma. An event that is challenging and exciting for one individual may be traumatic for another. The one for whom it is a mere challenge is able to "stay with it" and master it; the one who experiences it as a trauma is usually not.

By definition, then, a trauma contains repressed material. Contained in a trauma, too, are one or more intentions. At the very least, there is the intention to push it away, to blot it out, to repress it. And there are usually other intentions as well, such as the intention to fight back, to get revenge, to run away, or (quite commonly) the intention to make sure that nothing like this incident ever happens again.

An activity continues so long, and only so long, as the corresponding intention exists. That means that for each ongoing intention, there is an activity (at least a mental one) that continues as part of the here and now.

People subjectively define time in terms of the activity they are engaged in. Objectively, time is a featureless continuum. But subjectively, time is divided up into chunks—periods of time. For every given activity (and for every given intention) there is a corresponding period of time, and so long as you have an intention, you remain in the period of time defined by that intention (and activity). Holding onto an intention holds you in the period of time that commenced with the formulation of that intention. There are only two ways of ending an intention:

1. Fulfilling the intention, whereupon it ends spontaneously. You can't keep intending to win a race after you have won it.

2. Unmaking it. Even if you don't fulfill an intention, you can decide not to have that intention any more and cause it to end. This, however, requires a conscious decision. You have to be aware of the intention and why you formed it.

But what if the intention is buried in the middle of a repressed trauma? In this case, neither condition (1) nor (2) can be satisfied, and the intention persists indefinitely. The person remains in the period of time defined by that intention, i.e., within the traumatic incident. The incident floats on as part of present time and is easily triggered (i.e., the person is easily reminded of it, consciously or unconsciously).

The only way a person can exit from that period of time (and from the intentions, feelings and behaviors engendered by the trauma) is by confronting the incident, at which point the following becomes clear:

> a. What intentions were formulated at the time of the incident.
>
> b. Why they were formulated at that time.

Then, and only then, one can satisfy condition (2), above, for ending an intention, and one can let go of the intention. Without a thorough anamnesis, condition (2) cannot be satisfied.

8. How does TIR compare with other techniques for addressing traumatic stress?

Please see *Beyond Trauma: Conversations on Traumatic Incident Reduction, 2nd Ed* (2005).

9. What research exists to support the effectiveness of TIR?

In 1994, Charles Figley and Joyce Carbonell studied four different approaches to trauma resolution in their *Active Ingredient* study. Specifically, they observed TIR, Eye Movement Desensitization and Reprocessing (EMDR), Visual/Kinesthetic Dissociation (VK/D), and Thought Field Therapy (TFT). In their view, all are effective. However, their study was not designed as an outcome study. You can find a reprint of the Active Ingredient study in *TIR: Research and Results* (2005).

Lori Beth Bisbey completed a study of 57 victims of violent crime in February 1995. All of them suffered from

PTSD. The study compared TIR to both Direct Therapeutic Exposure (DTE) and waiting list controls, using a variety of test instruments. Waiting list controls showed no significant improvement over time; DTE showed significant improvement over controls (P < .01) on test instruments relating to PTSD; TIR performed significantly better than DTE (P < .01) on most test instruments. This study was part of her Ph.D. thesis and was done under the auspices of the California School of Professional Psychology, San Diego, CA.

Wendy Coughlin completed a study of TIR on Panic and Anxiety Disorders in May 1995. Her study concluded that "there was a substantial and statistically significant reduction in State Trait Anxiety for the entire sample. State Anxiety levels dropped by nearly one-third of their original levels. Based on the STAI scoring, the drop moved the group average from an anxiety level which would cause clinical concern and personal discomfort to a level that is considered normal for most people." This study was part of her Ph.D. thesis and was done under the auspices of Union Institute, Cincinnati, Ohio.

Pamela V. Valentine completed a study of TIR applied to 123 incarcerated females at the Federal Correction Institute in Tallahassee, Florida in 1997. Her work was presented at the Tenth National Symposium on Doctoral Research in Social Work in 1998. The study showed, after treatment using TIR, "...a statistically significant decrease in symptoms of posttraumatic stress disorder (and its related subscales and of depression and anxiety." This study was part of her Ph.D. thesis and was done under the auspices of Florida State University.

Summaries of all three studies as well as an outcome study on TIR with at-risk middle-school children can be found in the publication *Traumatic Incident Reduction: Research and Results*, Ed. By Victor R. Volkman.

10. How can I find out more about TIR?

Visit www.TIR.org

11. How can one get trained in TIR?

You can learn TIR by taking the first TIR Workshop (see www.TIRtraining.org) from a certified TIR trainer. Consult the Traumatic Incident Reduction Association website as above in order to find the nearest certified trainer.

12. What are the prerequisites for training?

A willingness and intention to help others and a reasonable degree of intelligence.

13. How can I refer people to a TIR practitioner?

Visit www.TIR.org

Appendix	Basics Concepts of Critical
B	Incident Stress Management By George Doherty

About the Author

George W. Doherty is President of the Rocky Mountain Region Disaster Mental Health Institute in Laramie, Wyoming (www.rmrinstitute.org). The Institute sponsors an annual Disaster Mental Health Conference as well as CISM training around the Wyoming area. Some of the following material has been excerpted from ICISF training materials and we acknowledge them for permission to use it here.

The ICISF and CISM

International Critical Incident Stress Foundation (ICISF) is a non-profit, open membership foundation dedicated to the prevention and mitigation of disabling stress through the provision of

- Education, training and support services for all Emergency Services professions;

- Continuing education and training in Emergency Mental Health Services for the Mental Health Community;

- and Consultation in the establishment of Crisis and Disaster Response Programs for varied organizations and communities worldwide.

George Everly and Jeffery Mitchell are located through the ICISF Headquarters in Ellicott City, MD. The mailing address is: ICISF, 3290 Pine Orchard Lane, Ellicott City, MD 21042

Important Definitions:
- **Critical Incident Stress Management** (CISM) (Everly & Mitchell, 1997, 1999; Everly & Langlieb, 2003) – Describes a comprehensive, phase sensitive and integrated, multi-component approach to crisis/disaster intervention.
- **Critical Incidents** are unusually challenging events that have the potential to create significant human distress and can overwhelm one's usual coping mechanisms.
- The psychological **Distress** in response to critical incidents such as emergencies, disasters, traumatic events, terrorism, or catastrophes is called a **Psychological Crisis** (Everly & Mitchell, 1999).
- Crisis intervention targets the *response*, not the *event*, per se. Thus, crisis intervention and disaster mental health interventions must be predicated upon assessment of need.
- **Psychological Crisis:** An acute *response* to a trauma, disaster, or other critical incident wherein:
  - o Psychological homeostasis (balance) is disrupted (increased stress)
  - o One's usual coping mechanisms have failed
  - o There is evidence of significant distress, impairment, dysfunction
    (adapted from Caplan, 1964, *Preventive Psychiatry*).

What Is Crisis Intervention?

Crisis Intervention is:
- An active, short-term, supportive, helping process.
- Acute intervention designed to mitigate the crisis response.
- Not psychotherapy or a substitute for psychotherapy.

The goals of Crisis Intervention are:

- Stabilization
- Symptom reduction
- Return to adaptive functioning, or
- Facilitation of access to continued care.

In addition to pre-incident preparation, crisis and disaster mental health intervention may be the best way to foster resiliency.

- **Resistance** refers to the ability of an individual, a group, an organization, or even an entire population, to literally *resist* manifestations of clinical distress, impairment, or dysfunction associated with critical incidents, terrorism, and even mass disasters. *Resistance* may be thought of as a form of psychological/ behavioral *immunity* to distress and dysfunction. Pre-incident training/ preparation may be best way to build resistance.

- **Resilience** refers to the ability of an individual, a group, an organization, or even an entire population, to rapidly and effectively rebound from psychological and/or behavioral perturbations associated with critical incidents, terrorism, and even mass disasters.

- **Recovery** refers to the ability of an individual, a group, an organization, or even an entire population, to literally *recover the ability to adaptively function,* both psychologically and behaviorally, in the wake of a significant clinical distress, impairment, or dysfunction subsequent to critical incidents, terrorism, and even mass disasters. Crisis intervention, treatment, and rehabilitation speeds recovery.

CISM is a strategic intervention system. It possesses numerous **tactical interventions**:

- Pre-incident education, preparation
- Assessment
- Strategic Planning
- Large Group Crisis Intervention:
  o Demobilizations (large groups of rescue/ recovery)
  o Respite/Rehab Sectors
  o Crisis Management Briefings (CMB)
- Small Group Crisis Intervention:
  o Defusings (small groups)
  o Small group CMB
  o "Debriefing" — Critical Incident Stress Debriefing (CISD)
  o One-on-one crisis intervention, including individual PFA
  o Family CISM
  o Organizational/ Community intervention, consultation
  o Pastoral crisis intervention
  o Follow-up and referral for continued care.

Core Competencies Of Comprehensive Crisis Intervention:

- Assessment/triage: benign vs. malignant symptoms
- Strategic planning and utilizing an integrated multi-component crisis intervention system within an incident command system
- One-on-one crisis intervention
- Small group crisis intervention
- Large group crisis intervention
- Follow-up and referral

The CISD and the entire field of CISM are not substitutes for psychotherapy. Rather, they are elements within the emergency mental health system designed to precede and complement psychotherapy, i.e., part of the full continuum of care.

What Are Critical Incidents?

A Critical Incident is any event that generates such intense emotional energy that it overwhelms an individual's or a group's ability to cope and causes impairment in work or personal activities. Some examples of Critical Incidents include:

- Suicide of a colleague
- Line of duty death
- Serious on-the-job injury
- Disaster or a multi-casualty incident
- Police shooting, or killing or wounding of any person in a routine operation, or any event with significant threat to those involved
- Significant events involving children
- Relatives of a known victim
- Prolonged incidents, especially with a loss
- Events with excessive media interest
- Any significant distressful event

Critical Incident Stress is the cognitive, physical, and emotional state of arousal that is part of the crisis response. Critical Incident Stress (CIS) is also known as "Post Traumatic Stress," which is not the same as PTSD. CIS is a normal response of normal people to an abnormal event.

What are the Signs And Symptoms Of Distress?

Distress may occur in any of several areas:
- Cognitive (Thinking)
- Emotional

- Behavioral
- Physical
- Spiritual

Posttraumatic Stress (PTS) is a normal survival response; Posttraumatic Stress Disorder (PTSD) is a pathologic variant of that normal survival reaction. PTSD results from violation of expectations and deeply held beliefs (i.e. worldviews).

Guidelines for Triage:

Refer for further evaluation any severe dysfunctions or impairment, but especially:

- Panic
- Enduring Cognitive Impairment
- Alternative Realities
- Vegetative Depression
- Hopelessness, Helplessness
- Self-destructive, other-destructive ideation, inclinations, actions (including antisocial acts)
- Violence, or threats of violence
- Guilt associated with depression
- Dissociation
- Psychogenic amnesia
- Potentially malignant physical reactions (bleeding, unconsciousness, numbness, paralysis, severe arrhythmias, etc.)
- Self-medication
- Whenever in doubt – refer

Role Of Psychological Therapy:

Crisis intervention and psychological therapy are opposite ends of the same continuum of care. Cognitive Behavioral Therapy (CBT), as a "psychological therapy," has shown great promise and is the current "treatment" of choice. Other psychotherapeutic models (e.g., EMDR) also seem applicable. This may be where TIR can also be included.

Keep CISD within the multi-component context of CISM: CISD should never be a stand-alone intervention. It should only be used when it is part of a package of interventions which includes follow-up services. The group CISD process should never be used for individuals since it was designed for groups. CISD should not be used to achieve psychotherapeutic outcome. CISD is neither psychotherapy nor a substitute for psychotherapy.

The majority of individuals exposed to a traumatic event will not need formal psychological intervention, beyond being provided relevant information. The focus should be upon the individual more than on the event. Assessment is essential. Assessment is an on-going dynamic process, rather than a discrete, static stage. Normalization of the crisis response is to be encouraged, but should never lead one to dismiss serious crisis reactions.

Unless the magnitude of impairment is such that the individual represents a threat to self or others, crisis intervention should be voluntary. The interventionist must be careful not to interfere with natural recovery or adaptive compensatory mechanisms.

The potential for vicarious traumatization must be reduced. Individuals should not be encouraged to talk about or relive the event, unless they are comfortable doing so. When in doubt, seek assistance, supervision.

Tactics and Strategy

The challenge in crisis intervention is not only developing TACTICAL skills in the "core intervention competencies," but is in knowing WHEN to best STRATEGICALLY employ the most appropriate TYPE of intervention for the situation. Consider when choosing the TYPE of intervention:

- THREAT: What specific "threat" is the focus of the intervention plan, e.g., hurricane, bioterrorism, earthquake, etc.?
- THEMES: Themes are factors that may serve to modify the psychological impact of the event or the nature of the intervention (child fatalities, mass disasters, biological contagion)
- TARGET: What target populations will most likely be in need of assistance/ support?
- TYPE: What specific types of interventions will be needed, e.g., demobilizations, town meetings, hotlines, CISDs, etc.?
- TIMING: When will each of the selected interventions be implemented so as to be most effective?
- TEAM: What resources will it take to provide the right interventions at the right time? Internal vs. external resources.

What is Demobilization?

Demobilization is usually a one time (end of shift; end of deployment), large-group information process for emergency services, military or other operations staff who have been exposed to a significant traumatic event such as a disaster or terrorist attack. The main functions of Demobilization are:

- Provide practical information (presentation in structured demobilization with handouts); [etc.]
- Provide a rest break after disaster work and before returning to home or non-disaster related duties (in both demobilizations and in respite).
- Opportunity for assessment of personnel to see who might need additional support (in both demobilizations and respite sectors).

- For large groups of emergency response personnel.
- After disaster or other large-scale incident.

The goals of Demobilization include:
- Psychological decompression
- Rest
- Refreshment
- Information
- Secondary psychological screening

Crisis Management Briefings:

Crisis Management Briefings are structured large group community/organizational "town meetings" designed to provide information about the incident, control rumors, educate about symptoms of distress, inform about basic stress management, and identify resources available for continued support, if desired. May be especially useful in response to community violence or terrorism. May have small group applications. (Everly, IJEMH, 2000).

Crisis Management Briefings (CMB) may be utilized with a traumatic event of any size that impacts a large number of people. It is applicable to a wide variety of school, business, church, industrial, organizational and community based populations. CMBs have military and emergency services applications as well. The goals of CMB are specific and well-defined:

- Provide information
- Provide a sense of leadership
- Reduce sense of chaos
- Enhance credibility
- Control rumors;
- Provide coping resources
- Engender cohesion, morale
- Re-establish a sense of community
- Psychological screening

The CMB may be one of the most effective tools available in the early response to terrorism, especially the multi-media CMB in response to bioterrorism. For Military and Emergency Services personnel, the CMB is useful when they are returning to a disaster site or combat zone for additional shifts or tours of duty.

Crisis Management Briefings are not a solution to everything. Specifically, they are:

- NOT a press conference. Media are not permitted.
- NOT psychotherapy.
- NOT a CISD.
- NOT a substitute for psychotherapy.
- NOT a focus group.
- NOT a solution group for ongoing problems in organizations or communities.

Defusings

Defusings are small group discussions following within 8 to 12 hours of a critical event. It is a specific 3-phase structure and should require less than an hour. Defusings work ideally with a homogenous, peer-facilitated group in a sequestered location. The goals of Defusing are:

- Normalization / lower tension.
- Set expectations, provide information.
- Discuss coping methods.
- Identify those who need additional support.

Depending on the preparation level, there may not be a set of pre-arranged questions. Instead, questions may be developed "on the spot". If a defusing goes too "deep", team members gently shift to more cognitive questions.

In situations where there is evidence of significant affective lability, overwhelming emotions, dysfunctional arousal, and/or group cohesion is fragile (hyper-reactive, divisive, evidence of anger or blame), CISD would be contraindicated.

Critical Incident Stress Debriefing (CISD):

CISD is a structured GROUP discussion concerning a critical incident, and as such it requires a team approach. It was first described by Mitchell (1983) for use with emergency services personnel. Historical roots are in military psychiatry. S.L.A. Marshall's Historical Event Reconstruction Debriefing (HERD) is one such example. Specifically, the goals of CISD are:

- Mitigate distress.
- Facilitate psychological normalization and psychological "closure" (reconstruction).
- Set appropriate expectations for psychological/ behavioral reactions.
- Serve as a forum for stress management education.
- Identify external coping resources.
- Serve as a platform for psychological triage and referral.

CISD follows a specific 7-phase structure:
- Introduction
- Fact Phase
- Thought Phase
- Reaction Phase
- Symptom Phase
- Teaching Phase
- Re-Entry Phase

Summary

CISM is a comprehensive, phase sensitive, and integrated, multi-component approach to crisis/disaster intervention.

While CISM approaches can be applied to work with victims, the primary mission is to provide this for first responders. It is also applied within organizations as an internal program. It is important to distinguish between "Traumatic Incident" and "Critical Incident". For example, a Critical Incident as defined by Mitchell (2006) and ICISF is "an unusually challenging event that has the potential to create significant human distress and can overwhelm one's usual coping mechanisms."

I would not place behavioral treatment under the medical model. The Behavioral Model deals with adjustment and adaptation and describes behavior as adaptive or functional. Behavioral Models tend to stay away from the term "mental illness" and rather define behaviors as adaptive or functional. It is the behavior that counts. Add the cognitive component and it involves things such as self-talk and self-verbal-reinforcement of observed as well as thinking behaviors. Behavior Therapy is usually goal-oriented—goals are defined by both the therapist and client collaboratively.

CISM is a strategic intervention system which contains numerous tactical interventions. The challenge in crisis intervention is not only developing TACTICAL skills in the "core intervention competencies", but is in knowing when to best STRATEGICALLY employ the most appropriate intervention for the situation.

The final stage of CISD is sometimes mistakenly called referral. The correct phase is termed "Re-entry". Phase six is a Teaching Phase in which referral information is provided as an available resource.

It is important to differentiate between Post Traumatic Stress (PTS) and Post Traumatic Stress Disorder (PTSD). PTS is a normal response to an abnormal, highly unusual situation. PTSD can result when symptoms do not resolve and continue over an extended period of time (see criteria listed in DSM-IV).

Table B-1: Summary of Commonly Used Crisis/ Disaster Interventions (adapted from Raphael, 1986; Everly & Langlieb, 2003; NIMH, 2002; Sheehan, et al., 2004; DHHS, 2004; Everly & Castellano, 2005; Everly & Parker, 2005; NOVA, 2002):

Intervention	Timing	Target Group	Potential Goals
1. Pre-event planning/ preparation	Pre-event	Anticipated target/victim population	Anticipatory guidance. Foster resistance, resilience
2. Assessment	Pre-intervention	Those directly & indirectly exposed	Determination of need for intervention
3. Indiv. Crisis Intervention (including "psych first aid")	As needed.	Individuals as needed.	Assessment Screening. Education. Normalization. Reduction of Acute distress Triage: facilitation of continued support.
4. Demobilization	Shift disengagement. End of deployment.	Emergency personnel. Large groups.	Decompression. Screening. Triage. Education. Ease transition
5. Respite Sector	On-going large-scale events.	Emergency personnel. Large groups.	Respite. Refreshment. Screening. Triage Support.
6. Large Group CMB & Large group psych first aid	As needed.	Heterogenous large groups.	Inform. Control rumors. Increase cohesion.
7. "Group Debriefing" (CISD, PD, GCI, MSD, CED, HERD	Post-event... ~1-10 days acute incidents; ~3-4 weeks post mass disaster recovery phase	Small homogenouse groups w/equal trauma exposure. Often workgroups, emergency services, or military	Ventilation. Information. Normalization. Reduce acute distress. Increase cohesion, resilience. Screening. Triage. Follow-up is essential

...Continued on next page

Intervention	Timing	Target Group	Potential Goals
8. Defusing (and small group psych first aid)	On-going events & post-event (<12 hrs) may be repeated	Small homogenous groups. May be similar to HERD in process	Stabilization. Ventilation. Reduce acute distress. Screening. Information. Increase cohesion, resilience
9. Small Group Crisis Management Briefing (sCMB)	On-going events & Post-event) May be repeated	Small groups seeking info. c/o delving into affect.	Information. Control rumors. Reduce acute distress. Increase cohesion, resilience. Screening/triage.
10. Family Crisis Intervention	Pre-event & as needed.	Families	Consists of a wide array of interventions including pre-event prep, indiv. interventions, sCMB, "debriefing" etc.
11. Organizational/Leadership Consultation	Pre-event & as needed.	Organizations affected by trauma or disaster	Improve organizational preparedness & response.
12 Pastoral Crisis Intervention:	As needed.	Those who desire faith-based presence/crisis intervention, e.g. Ministry of presence. Religious intervention, if desired.	Faith-based support, e.g. information, advocacy, liason.
13. Follow-up, Referral	As needed.	Intervention recipients and those exposed	Assure continuity of care.
14. Strategic planning	Pre-event & during	Anticipated exposed/victim populations	Improve overall disaster MH response

Appendix	TIR Rules of Facilitation and
C	Communication Skills (condensed)
	By Frank A. Gerbode, M.D.

Much of the skill of a Traumatic Incident Reduction facilitator has nothing to do with one's knowledge of post-traumatic stress disorder or of the theory or technique of TIR. The facilitator's greatest challenge is to create an environment suitable for viewing and to conduct the session according to the rules governing the procedure.

The Rules of Facilitation were written to help the facilitator of a viewing session bring each session to a successful conclusion, that is, a successful conclusion according to the viewer.

The Rules of Facilitation empower the viewer to be independent, instead of dependent on the facilitator.

Considering how important these rules are in a session, think for a moment what life would be like if we adapted these rules to our day-to-day interactions with others.

1. **Ensure that the viewer is in optimum physical condition for the viewing session.** This means that a viewing session is not delivered to someone who is hungry, tired, physically ill, or under the influence of alcohol or psychoactive drugs (except when drugs are prescribed as a medical necessity). Sometimes viewing is delivered to a person who is not in optimum condition because that seems like the only way the person may ever get to an optimum condition. However, a viewer in a non-optimum condition has to work harder in session.

2. **Ensure that the session is being given in a suitable place and at a suitable time.** Ensure that the viewing environment is secure, private, clean, quiet, and

environmentally comfortable. Also make sure that the time is safe, that is, enough session time is set aside for the viewer to reach a good end point for the session. Make sure all cell phones, pagers, and desk phones are turned off.

3. **Do not interpret for the viewer.** Do not tell the viewer anything about the material being viewed, including what it means or how to think or feel about it. Facilitators differ radically from therapists, who may offer interpretation and advice to the client. When a therapist is delivering a Metapsychology viewing session, he informs the client that he will be operating under a different set of rules.

4. **Do not evaluate for the viewer.** Avoid indicating, in any way, that what the viewer has said or done is right or wrong. Do not judge, criticize, disparage, or invalidate the viewer or her perceptions, assumptions, conclusions, values, reactions, thoughts, feelings, or actions. Also, do not validate the viewer because such praise may lead her to sense a judgmental atmosphere and to anticipate that the next judgment might not be so favorable.

5. **Control the session and take complete responsibility for it without dominating the viewer.** This makes it unnecessary for the viewer to be concerned about what comes next in the viewing procedure and allows total attention to be placed on the viewing.

6. **Be sure to comprehend what the viewer is saying.** A viewer knows right away when the facilitator does not comprehend and then feels alone and unsupported. The facilitator who does not comprehend must seek clarification and, at the same time, take responsibility for the need to do so. The facilitator might say, "I'm sorry. I didn't get what you said. Could you give it to me again", and would not say, "You are being unclear," or even, "Please clarify what you mean."

7. **Be interested in the viewer and in what the viewer is saying instead of being interesting to the viewer.** A viewer generally knows immediately whether or not the facilitator is really interested. If the facilitator becomes interesting, the viewer's attention will be pulled away from the viewing itself. The facilitator's interest supports the viewer's willingness to view and report on the material being viewed.

8. **Act in a predictable way so as not to surprise or distract the viewer.** It is not appropriate for a facilitator to disclose personal feelings during a viewing session. The viewer has enough to do when confronting his personal issues without having to deal with extraneous actions, remarks, or displays of emotion on the part of the facilitator.

9. **Do not try to work with someone against that person's will or in the presence of any protest.** Sometimes a relative, friend or employer will succeed in persuading a person to do viewing when she does not really want to. In such a circumstance, viewing does not work well or at all. Accordingly, the facilitator must be guided only by the viewer's interest and priorities and must never try to coerce or manipulate the viewer into running a particular procedure when the viewer is not really interested in doing so. The facilitator must never rush the viewer. The viewer who senses that a quick response is being demanded will not take time to do the major beneficial action in viewing, the act of viewing itself.

10. **Carry each viewing action to a success for the viewer.** Be certain not to end a viewing procedure at a point of failure or incompleteness. This is the main reason sessions must not be fixed in length. One of the major functions of a facilitator is to help the viewer find the courage and confidence to confront difficult material that he has not been willing or able to confront alone. When viewing becomes painful, difficult, or embarrassing, the

viewer may feel like ending the session. Should this occur, the facilitator's job is to encourage the viewer to stick with it and to confront and handle the difficulty to a point of resolution. Fortunately, viewing procedures are sufficiently powerful and effective to warrant such confidence on the part of an experienced facilitator.

11. **Maintain a firm and primary intention to help the viewer.** As obvious as it may seem, a facilitator who is mainly interested in improving clinical skills or in making money, even if he also intends to help the viewer, will tend to lose a viewer's trust. In order to maintain the level of viewer/facilitator confidence required to preserve the viewer's sense of session security, the viewer's interests must be preserved at all times. The facilitator must agree not to reveal or use anything the viewer says for any purpose except to help the viewer and to enhance the process of viewing.

Although some of these Rules may seem obvious or simplistic, particularly to trained therapists, they need to be enumerated because they are essential to the overall method that supports the work of successful TIR-related techniques.

Communication Skills

The following are Communication Skills as taught in the Traumatic Incident Reduction Workshop. These are also colloquially known as the Communication Exercises (CEs for short) as there is a specific exercise involved to develop each corresponding skill:

1. **Being Present:** is to be comfortably present in front of a viewer with your attention in present time and without having to do anything.

2. **Confronting:** is to be able to face things or people without flinching or avoiding them, simply being fully aware of them, paying attention to them, being present with them, and not necessarily having to do anything to them or about them.

3. **Interest:** is directed attention.

4. **Delivery:** is to deliver a specific viewing question or instruction clearly.

5. **Acknowledgments:** are to either end a communication or to encourage further communication.

6. **Encouraging communication:** elicits further communication.

7. **Getting your questions answered:** Addressing client concern disrelated to what is being handled and bring the client back to completing what was started.

Index

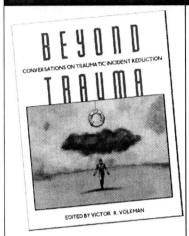

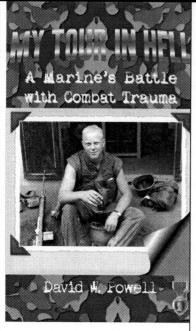
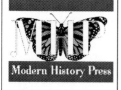

Printed in the United States
74328LV00014BA/227